POWER HERBS

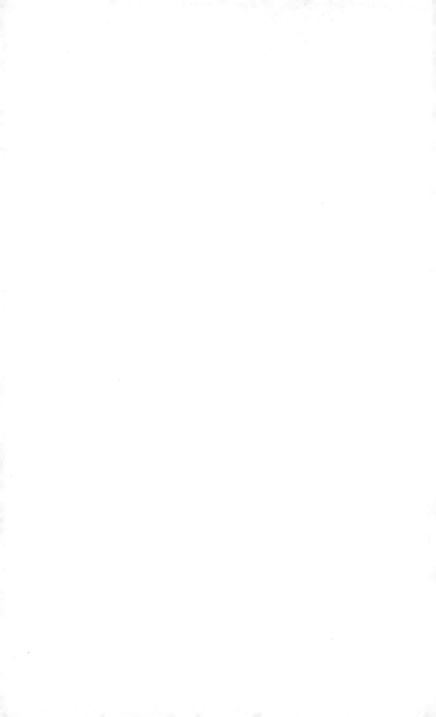

POWER
HERBS

A PRACTICAL GUIDE TO

FIFTY HEALING HERBS FROM

THE EAST AND WEST

LOUIS J. VANRENEN

JEREMY P. TARCHER/PUTNAM

A MEMBER OF PENGUIN PUTNAM INC.

NEW YORK

Jeremy P. Tarcher/Putnam
a member of
Penguin Putnam Inc.
375 Hudson Street
New York, NY 10014
www.penguinputnam.com

Library of Congress Cataloging-in-Publication Data
Vanrenen, Louis J.
Power herbs: a practical guide to fifty healing herbs from the
East and West / Louis J. Vanrenen.
p.   cm.
Includes bibliographical references.
ISBN 1-58542-033-6
1. Herbs—Therapeutic use.   I. Title.
RM666.H33 V364   2000   99-087667
615'.321—dc21

Printed in the United States of America
1   3   5   7   9   10   8   6   4   2

This book is printed on acid-free paper. ∞

Book design by Chris Welch

THIS BOOK IS DEDICATED TO
JOHNNA ALBI (1946 – 1995).

PREFACE

This guidebook to major medicinal plants is to be used as an adjunct to regular medical care, whether by a conventional physician, homeopathic doctor, naturopath, professional herbalist, or acupuncturist.

This book, based on two decades of study, research, and clinical practice, is founded on the principles of Oriental medicine, Western research, homeopathy, European herbalism, and American Indian medicine.

Thanks to the colleagues and teachers who have supported and guided me over the past quarter of a century, and to those luminaries who have inspired me, including: Dr. William Boericke, Dr. Harvey W. Felter, Dr. Richard Evans Shultes, and many others.

In addition, gratitude to my agent, Marlene Finn Gabriel, my secretary, Sharon Irving, and Ariana and Gabriel, my children.

CONTENTS

THE REBIRTH OF HERBAL MEDICINE

I n America, herbal remedies have had an astonishing resurgence during the 1990s, along with ancient healing systems like acupuncture and massage. Not long ago herbs were relegated to the back shelf of mainstream consciousness, a quaint relic from the past only popular with the "health nuts" and the like. The situation appears to have changed dramatically, but in fact interest in herbs has been growing steadily the past forty years, as more people have become interested in the welfare of our bodies and planet. With the growing interest in health promotion and disease prevention, it is now seen that herbal remedies are the nearly perfect vehicle: gentle, nourishing, and, if used intelligently, safer, in fact much safer, than the potent prescription drugs. Many herbal medicines can be seen as medicinal foods, rich with vitamins and minerals and profoundly nourishing for the body and person.

People are not well informed about herbs. Every day people are buying herbs, spending millions of dollars, and using them for colds, flu, fatigue, depressions, energy, sex drive, relaxation, and many of the other daily problems that bedevil busy modern people. They are going out in huge numbers all across the nation to buy the famous herbs like St. John's wort, echinacea, and ginseng — remedies that have received a remarkable level of publicity in recent years. Often they buy on the advice of an article, a television ad, or a whim and do not really know what they are taking, how much, even why. Most often they are too embarrassed to ask their doctors; if they did, their doctors might not know how to respond, though more and more doctors are now familiar with herbs.

What are herbs good for? Are they effective and safe? How do I take them? There is no doubt that millions of Americans want to know more about the major herbs on the market today. This book is a resource intended to serve this growing interest in natural medicines for patients, individuals, and families.

While the passion for herbs might be new in late-twentieth-century America, this is not true for the rest of the planet. In third world nations, where the bulk of the world's populace live, herbs remain a staple, an integral part of people's culture and heritage. In modern countries like Italy, France, and Germany, herbs never lost their luster in the transition to technological medicine; Europe has a durable tradition of natural medicine.

In 1991 a dramatic discovery emerged from a melting

glacier in northern Italy: two hikers discovered a well-preserved mummy, the now famous Ice Man, who died about 5,300 years ago. Seven years later this find continues to fascinate scientists from different disciplines. Not only could this man's remains be studied, but the remnants of tools and clothes, an astonishing discovery, had also survived the thousands of years. The Ice Man, who presumably died while crossing a mountain pass, could provide the modern world with many clues about life in the Stone Age. One of these clues revolved around the use of medicine in those very distant times.

The assumption has been that Stone Age people had at best a primitive understanding of medicine and healing. One of the clues that survived with the Ice Man were two mysterious spheres threaded on leather thongs. Originally thought to be tinder for starting fires, they are now said to be the woody fruit of a tree fungus that has therapeutic properties. Not only is the fungus a laxative, but it also contains oils that are toxic to intestinal parasites. Professor Luigi Capasso of Italy's National Archeological Museum reported in the British medical journal *Lancet* that Ice Man was, most likely, able to recognize the nature of his illness and use an herbal remedy that was remarkably specific for his condition. The professor reported: "We have no other finding in this condition of comparable antiquity for Europe." He also speculates that tattoos on the Ice Man's skin are evidence of localized treatment for muscle pain — even, I suggest, a basic form of acupuncture.

Dr. David Pilbeam, a Harvard anthropologist, is a specialist in Paleolithic cultures and certainly well qualified to comment on Dr. Capasso's discoveries. Modern Western science has rigidly assumed that "primitive" humans were abysmally ignorant, particularly about such arcane subjects as medical diagnosis. Dr. Pilbeam suggests that we need to examine these assumptions and even prejudices. He says: "People have empirical minds. Western culture tends to underestimate the knowledge of other cultures and other times."[1] Indeed, medical history is filled with unexamined facts. The ancient Chinese, for example, applied molds, which are now known to contain antibiotics, on skin infections. In fact, the whole herbal pharmacopoeia of the Orient contains hundreds of therapeutic plants still very much in use today. American Indians utilized plants now known to contain antitumor properties on skin cancers. One American Indian medicine, May apple (*Podophyllum peltatum*), is now converted into a drug for modern cancer therapy. For hundreds of years African and American Indian medicine men and women have been using effective medicines for disease prevention and treatment. Furthermore, many systems of traditional healing, while lacking the benefits of modern technological medicine, are based on principles of ecology and holism.

Our distant friend the Ice Man provides clues to the earliest rational use of herbal medicine, but since his time people around the globe have used herbal medicine for thousands of years. Today, around the world 80 percent of the world's people still use herbal medicines in one way or another. Complex, sophisticated systems of herbal medicine, most notably from China and India, are still flourishing in their own societies. What's more, thousands of Americans and

1. *Boston Globe*, December 14, 1998.

Europeans are now benefiting from these venerable systems and turning to herbal medicine in vast numbers.

What is especially interesting is that in two of the more scientifically advanced countries in the world, Germany and Japan, herbal medicines are very much alive, in fact booming. It is estimated that 70 percent of Japanese physicians now make some use of their traditional herbal system, *Kampo*, or refer patients to herbal specialists. Many of the early discoveries in the extraction of drugs from plants came from Germany, in the last century, so it is not an exaggeration to say that modern pharmaceutical medicine started in that nation. Paradoxically, herbal medicine is also a living and durable tradition in Germany; many herbal remedies are popular there with doctors and people. Much of the recent research in herbal medicines comes from Germany, where they are studied, respected, regulated, and approved as over-the-counter drugs. Recently the German Commission E, a government medical association, published a major clinical guide to herbal medicine. This book, which examines the medicinal uses of numerous medicinal plants, marks a major turning point in the use of natural medicines in the West.

Ironically, many great American natural medicines are respected in Europe, while in America they continue to languish as they have for one hundred years. It is somewhat astonishing that conventional American medicine is still so lagging in the study and clinical use of herbal medicines. Dr. Varro Tyler, dean emeritus of the School of Pharmacy at Purdue University and a leading American authority on medicinal plants, echoed a theme that runs through this book when he said: "So many of our good American plant drugs (such as echinacea and saw palmetto) had to be researched in Europe because we don't have reasonable laws and regulations here that promote the scientific development of botanicals. I personally think that's just an utter tragedy."[2]

However, after much foot-dragging, herbal medicines are now receiving research support, and the claims and medicines of many generations can be thoroughly examined. Scientifically and publicly, herbal medicines are regaining their credibility, a development that is long overdue.

What qualifies me to offer this guide? I have had over twenty years of experience with herbal medicines from four different but interrelated perspectives: (1) I have grown medicinal plants for twenty-five years; (2) I have hunted for them in diverse forests, jungles, and fields; (3) as a health professional I have had extensive experience with the clinical use of herbal medicines; and (4) I have studied these plants, particularly the therapeutic properties of the various constituents. The scientific examination of healing foods and plants has literally exploded in the past decade, making for a fascinating field of research and offering the opportunity, for the first time in our history, to understand herbs from a historical, clinical, and biochemical point of view. We live in an exciting era.

---

2. Jean Carper, *Miracle Cures* (New York: HarperCollins, 1997).

PART ONE

HERBAL MEDICINES AROUND THE WORLD

THE GOAL OF THIS BOOK

The heart of this book is an introduction to fifty herbal medicines from around our planet. Thousands of medicinal plants exist on this planet; I have distilled these down to fifty that I consider the most useful for the average person. Half of these remedies are from Asia and other parts of the globe, but their names, for the most part, are no longer exotic. The major natural remedies from Europe, America, and Asia are now becoming global, as the two halves of the globe share information. In America there is a renewed interest in herbal and natural healing, not only for first aid and home use but also for disease prevention. Indeed, one of the main advantages of modern herbs is their ability to improve health without side effects.

Power Herbs is not for those who want to identify, grow, or prepare their own herbal medicines—complex endeavors. Today, herbal medicines are very popular, and there is a bewildering array of natural remedies on the market. In pharmacies and health food stores, the everyday customer is confused by the many commercial preparations: capsules, extracts, formulas, and tablets. This book is intended to help people use the best of these commercial preparations, which are easy to use, convenient, and effective.

Power Herbs is not intended for serious health conditions; it is to be used for simple everyday problems, as well as for health maintenance and to promote longevity. In fact, I strongly advise that people use herbal medicines with respect and always take advantage of professional help. This practical handbook is offered with great respect for the value of regular medicine, doctor's visits, and medical testing and is not intended to replace the judicious use of medical doctors and other health practitioners but to supplement their useful and necessary care.

What to do when you are run-down and tired, and holidays are coming up? Herbal remedies can increase energy and alleviate unpleasant symptoms without harming the body.

What to do when Johnny is coming down with a cold or flu? Natural medicines can be of assistance here and without the side effects of synthetic drugs.

What to do when granny has had a hip operation and is still experiencing some stiffness and pain? Natural remedies can alleviate the pain and hasten the healing.

Herbal remedies can also promote better health and even

create a longer life. These positive effects are not an exaggeration. Centuries of experience and modern research are combining to validate the health value of these durable medicines. The reader will find here hundreds of fascinating therapeutic facts.

WHY NATURAL REMEDIES?

Natural remedies work. They are safe, nontoxic, and ecologically sound for the body and the environment. They are relatively easy to use, economical, and exciting to learn about. They are part of our heritage on this planet. Whether we are African American, Indian, Caucasian, Hispanic, or Jewish, our ancestors have used them for hundreds of years.

Many people are now realizing that the ecology of the human body is intimately connected to the ecology and health of the planet. Just as we do not want to bombard our water and earth with chemical drugs, so we do not want to fill our bodies with toxic substances. In the modern era the practical value of these herbs is increasingly supported by scientific research. In fact, recent decades have seen a global avalanche of studies and research confirming the value of medicinal plants and foods.

HOW DO HERBS DIFFER FROM PRESCRIPTION DRUGS?

For the most part herbal medicines are nourishing—filled with nutrients and antioxidants—as well as having specific therapeutic uses. Because they are a "whole" food, they are safer and less toxic than prescription drugs. Toxic herbal plants do exist, but they are not generally made into herbal medicines, except as a prescription item. Of course, there are a few herbal medicines that if taken in excess could make you sick, but this kind of irrational abuse leads to the same results with many foods. (Nonetheless, many herbs are medicinal and should be used with respect, and a few are best left to health professionals.)

Because nature owes the "patent" on natural remedies, there is little financial incentive for pharmaceutical companies to research and market them. Almost all prescription drugs are simply highly specific constituents that have been extracted from plants or chemical compounds. They are processed chemicals, often patented, with no nutrient value, and actually foreign to the evolution of life on this planet. Because they are potent chemicals they exert a powerful effect on the body, sometimes to very good purpose, but many also trigger side effects, even dangerous ones. This book promotes a global system of medicine, often called complementary, that aims to align so-called alternative medicines with modern technological medicine.

Herbal medicines can safely strengthen the body's healing responses and improve health as well as cure diseases. Therefore, their economy and practical value, their benefit for people of all ages and races, and the alleviation of suffering that they provide ensures their place in the scope of modern medicine. The healing potency and versatility of the fifty power herbs examined in this book does indeed support the title *Power Herbs*.

THE WESTERN HERBAL TRADITION

In the modern West, herbal and natural remedies have largely been associated with folk medicine, superstition, and old-fashioned practices. While it is true that in peasant societies the practice of herbal remedies was often riddled with folk fables, major systems of herbal medicine have existed on most continents for thousands of years. These systems, for example the Oriental system, contain great wisdom and medicines. Furthermore, the application and efficacy of the plant medicines is more successful than modern pundits could possibly imagine. Herbal medicine has existed in Europe for thousands of years, extending back to the Greeks, Romans, and Egyptians, even into the shadows of prehistory. In the ancient Greco-Roman world, healing was far more than the administration of medicines and, as in other cultures, involved foods, herbs, various kinds of bodywork, rituals, prayer, soothsaying, even dream interpretation. Hippocrates, often called the father of modern medicine, was the preeminent physician of ancient Greece. He wrote much about the medicinal qualities of food and plants. He also began the separation of medicine from magic and religion and started what we today consider the rational study and treatment of disease. Nonetheless, Hippocrates' medical philosophy was based on the idea of maintaining the balance of the whole person—body, emotions, and mind—thus preserving health. It was the duty of the physician to support the wisdom and healing powers of the body with as little harm as possible, a maxim that the Greek physicians shared with their Oriental counterparts—

and a theme that underlies the practice of much of herbal medicine throughout history. From time to time we see this principle popping back up in different guises: in naturopathy, homeopathy, acupuncture, and other practices.

In the ancient world one of the most accurate observers of plant medicines was the Greek Dioscorides, who wrote his classic work, *De Materia Medica*, in Latin, based on his decades of practical experience. Dioscorides, an army physician, traveled with the Roman troops in the first century A.D. This remarkable physician and herbalist carefully observed the plant world, studied all the sources available to him, and utilized his own experience to compile the most complete book of plant medicines in the ancient world. The Romans took good care of their far-ranging soldiers and employed many fine physicians like Dioscorides who had encyclopedic knowledge of countless medicinal plants and many complex formulas.

With the collapse of the Roman Empire, the scholarly examination of medicinal plants was left to the creative Arabs, who continued a rich tradition of learning through the Middle Ages. During the late Middle Ages and the dawn of the modern era, medical practice in Europe was a curious mixture of various practices and philosophies. Monasteries, with their superb herbal gardens, were often a reliable source of simple medicines, and indeed the monks kept alive a strong tradition of natural healing. Of course, the midwives, country herbalists, and traveling healers were always part of the scene, and these simple folk greatly relied on the medicines of the land. But little was done to thoroughly expand and classify the herbal medicines available to people of the time, and most books that came out after the birth of the printing press were not very accurate or dependable.

In the sixteenth and seventeenth centuries regular medical practice in the West was based on rigid obeisance to old Greco-Roman texts, most often preserved and handed on by the Arabs. Little attention was given to local medicines or to careful observation of plants, nature, or people; in fact, the regular physicians rarely used the simple herbs but instead relied on complex and expensive formulas of plant, mineral, and animal medicine. Some of the most famous medicines contained up to seventy-two ingredients, many of them awfully strange: exotic powders made from toads and snakes, minerals like coral and arsenic, even various kinds of excrement. Even worse was the growing reliance on toxic metals like mercury and antimony, used in preposterous quantities and sure to have killed literally thousands of unsuspecting patients. Along with bloodletting, physicians (and patients) wanted to see action in their medicine, thus the labeling of this era as heroic. Patients were purged with powerful drugs, bled, and blistered; in fact, they were often lucky to survive the expensive treatment. As with politicians today, public confidence in doctors plummeted. Doctors became the butt of cartoonists and satirists. The famous French playwright Molière amused his audiences with scathing satires about physicians. When asked by a curious Louis XIV about how he got along with his own doctor, Molière responded: "Sire, we chat; he prescribes remedies for me: I take no notice: and I get better."

The stagnant state of conventional medical arts really did not change much until the beginning of the twentieth century, but along the way European medicine experienced the stormy influence of medical pioneers: Paracelsus (1493–1546) and, in seventeenth-century London, the university-trained apothecary Nicholas Culpeper. Like Paracelsus, Culpeper called for a simple medicine for the people based on careful observation of people and nature. He published his *English Physician* in 1653, having written it, much to the horror of the contemporary doctors and apothecaries, in the language of the layperson. Culpeper, who had a classical medical training, was an extraordinary thorn in the side of the establishment. In his books, which offered a piquant mixture of useful facts and charming fable, he praised the value of hundreds of common herbs and described how the ordinary person might use them. In his London apothecary he was happy to treat the poor for little or no money, a fact that forever endeared him to the common folk of London.

Though we tend to deride Culpeper's work in modern times because of his astrological beliefs, his understanding of herbal medicines was quite reliable. There is no doubt that herbal medicine could, at times, be mixed up with fantasy and superstition, but Culpeper and many country folk, then as now, had a strong practical streak. They often knew specific qualities and functions of herbs for disease syndromes. This practice of using herbs from careful observation and long-term experience can be seen functioning today in the superb Oriental herbal system, which is literally based on hundreds of years of experience with millions of people. In the modern era, we do not appreciate the accumulated value of experience, observation, and intuition, the foundation of all traditional systems of natural healing.

One of Culpeper's quarrels with the fancy London physicians of his day was that they relied too much on exotic foreign medicines, metals, and ridiculously complex formulas. Time and time again, he asked, "Why not use the local medicines of England?" The regular physician, however, knew little about the local plants and herbal medicines, a situation that has remained unchanged to this day. In fact, doctors were notorious for scorning the simple country herbalists and mid-wives, and sometimes, when they felt threatened, they would do their best to put them in prison. It is sad to say that a common thread through the history of herbal medicine in the Western world has been an abiding prejudice against the simple natural medicines, the women healers, and the practice of medicine by "aliens"—Jews, gypsies, Indians, and Asians. Isolated physicians have repeatedly stood up against this tide of bias—men like Paracelsus, Samuel Hahnemann, and Culpeper—only to be ignored at best, at worst, silenced.

While Culpeper's message was heeded by many common folk, the established medicine drifted toward a greater reliance on the new wonder drugs, mercury and antimony—two dreaded poisons—as well as excessive bloodletting and purging. The European style of aggressive medicine was transported to America. One of the most famous physicians of colonial America, Benjamin Rush, was an avid bleeder; his main drug was the highly toxic calomel, made from mercury. The more aggressive the therapy, the more Dr. Rush was pleased. Sometimes pints of blood would be repeatedly bled from the unfortunate patient, and then the purgatives and poisons poured down his or her throat. George Washington died after being administered this "heroic" style of medicine after catching a flu; the poor man was bled copiously, poisons were poured down his throat, and one can only imagine that his beleaguered body was happy to pass on.

A signer of the constitution and probably the most influential doctor in America in his time, Dr. Rush exemplified the disdain that many conventional physicians have toward natural and botanical medicine. Like many white colonialists, he held a deep, abiding prejudice against Indians and did not think that their medicines amounted to anything. The bountiful natural pharmacy of America's prolific earth remained in the hands of the skilled Indian healers and the occasional white man or woman who was willing to learn from the "savages." As many visitors noticed in America, those Indians who were living free in their natural habit were remarkably healthy and robust. Many settlers, pioneers, hunters, and trappers who had to resort to the indigenous medicine were often suitably impressed. A notable handful of observers recognized that the Indian had a profound knowledge of healing and natural medicines. Some of these rare commentators had to come from overseas. John Wesley, founder of Methodism, visited America in the 1730s and observed that the Indians had "exceedingly few" diseases and their medicines were "quick and generally infallible."

The American natural medicines, the gift of our land, are still neglected in modern times. Many of the Indian medicines, however, are now becoming celebrities in the renaissance of natural and herbal medicine. Echinacea, the Sioux medicine for snakebites and wounds, is now a major natural medicine in Europe, as well as goldenseal and black cohosh. However, it is sad to say that the echo of prejudice exists: American Indian medicines are still not adequately studied, while exotic imports or chemical drugs are given high priority and massive funding.

In America during the last century, herbal medicine lived on in the country and ethnic communities. There was, however, a small coterie of physicians who respected indigenous natural medicines. There were several groups of this early "alternate" medical movement; in the nineteenth century the most prominent was called the Eclectic school. The Eclectics, originally inspired by the remarkable physician Wooster Beech, began their work as a reaction to the current "heroic" medicine that relied on mercury, strong purgatives, and bleeding. This group of "reform" physicians, centered in the Midwest, prided themselves on their respect for the natural healing powers of the body—Hippocrates' *vis medicatrix naturae*—and aimed to employ medicines that did not harm the body. They borrowed freely from the American Indian medicines. Dr. Beech, though trained at university, also studied with a venerable old "root doctor" who used the local medicines of the land. Members of Dr. Beech's medical reform movement called themselves the Eclectics because they claimed to take the best from different schools. From careful observation, research, and clinical experience, the Eclectics compiled some excellent books about natural medicines. Perhaps the culmination of their work was a book published in 1922 during the twilight of the Eclectic era, *The Eclectic Materia Medica*. It was written by a Dr. Harvey Wickes Felter and is quoted quite frequently in this book. Dr. Felter wrote intelligently about many of the modern power herbs.

At the end of the 1900s, the Eclectics began a thorough scientific investigation of herbs that, sadly, died out a few years later. Chemical drugs became completely dominant, and herbal medicines fell into disuse. Eclectics were considered a part of the past, relegated to history, and by 1920 only one or two of their schools existed in America. Today, however, modern herbalists respect their work and efforts. Many of the great American herbal medicines, now increasing in popularity, were first examined and used by the Eclectics. Their influence permeates this book, and their legacy has been revived in the naturopathic medical colleges, where one of the major courses includes herbal medicine. Sadly, conventional medical schools teach little about herbal and natural medicines, though there is now evidence that this situation is changing.

Another influence in modern herbology is homeopathy, a system of natural medicine that also flourished in nineteenth-century America. Homeopathy, based on the law of similars, uses minute doses of remedies to stimulate the healing force of the body. Many homeopathic remedies are made from herbs, but it is not herbal medicine. It is based on its own distinct principles. Developed in the early part of the nineteenth century by a German physician, Dr. Samuel Hahnemann, homeopathy spread rapidly through Europe as a sane alternative to the toxic drugging and bleeding of regular doctors. While homeopathy has had its ups and downs during the twentieth century, it has been increasing in popularity in America in recent decades. It is now practiced all over our planet, but because of its profound holistic principles, it has yet to be recognized by conventional medicine. Homeopathy, a medical discipline, is not in any way opposed to modern science and medical testing, and all over this planet homeopathic doctors are first trained in conventional medicine.

One of the great homeopaths of the turn of the century, William Boericke, was a physician greatly interested in the herbal medicines of America and Europe. In his classic book of medicinal substances, his *Materia Medica* of 1927, he included many American Indian medicines, as well as most of the great herbal medicines of Europe. Homeopathy, however, suffered a serious but temporary eclipse in the dawning age of wonder drugs and technological medicine, and for fifty years natural American medicines fell into decline, used only by a minority of Hispanics, Indians, and country folk.

In the first part of the twentieth century, remarkable advances revolutionized medical science, resulting in countless benefits in public health, diagnosis, and drugs. Furthermore, plants and chemicals could be analyzed and broken down to basic constituents and even synthetically re-created. The brave new world of chemical drugs hypnotized America, and the standard medical view was that herbal medicine was a remnant of a past we would prefer to forget. The magic bullet theory governed conventional medicine, so much so that it was forgotten that disease exists in the terrain of a person. Today, we are beginning to see that medicine is not as simple as finding the bullet for every disease. But in many ways it did seem that the era of "scientific" medicine had triumphed over disease with its many great discoveries and advances. Along the way, however, something crucial was overlooked: the healing power of the body—the *vis medicatrix naturae* of Hippocrates—and the ecological understanding of medicine based on the natural remedies of nature. Like Prometheus, modern man thought he could do better, far better, than clumsy nature.

This situation began to change in the 1960s as young people returned to nature, as people became disillusioned with the complete reliance on synthetic drugs, and as people began to see that the ecology of the Earth included the body as well. Another influence was the increasing openness to the study and appreciation of other cultures, particularly those of the American Indian and of Asia. These rich and vibrant cultures had, over many centuries, developed a respect for the body and its relation to nature and as a result had produced profound systems of ecological medicine based primarily on plant medicines and natural cures. In the 1960s and 1970s a few intrepid younger doctors and scholars even traveled to China and Japan and began to bring back the philosophy and practice of Oriental medicine, most notably the plant medicines and acupuncture.

When I began to study acupuncture, herbs, and Oriental medicine in 1976, I was considered unusual by friends and relatives. Herbal medicine and acupuncture were fringe practices at that time, considered the territory of eccentrics and Oriental aficionados. Twenty-two years later this attitude has changed dramatically. In 1998 acupuncture and herbal medicine are practiced in every state of the union, and herbs are available in most towns and cities. As several studies have clearly indicated, millions of Americans have turned to "alternate" treatments, including herbal medicine, to supplement conventional medicine. It is no exaggeration to say that herbal medicine is enjoying a rebirth in America after a brief hiatus of sixty or seventy years. In the 1990s the development of natural medicines reached a new pinnacle, supported by scientific research—much of it from Europe and Asia—and fertilized by global concerns and influences.

EASTERN AND ORIENTAL MEDICINE

Oriental medicine is an ancient tradition that is flourishing in the modern world for two major reasons: it uses superb natural remedies founded on centuries of clinical experience, and it derives from profound holistic principles. In Asia the system of natural medicine includes herbs, foods, varied massage techniques, acupuncture, and other methods. The herbal tradition is thousands of years old and utilizes hundreds of medicines from plants and minerals. Within this great multiplicity and fund of knowledge, there are about thirty truly great herbal medicines that can be confidently utilized by most Americans.

The major herbal tradition in the modern world comes from China, where a continuous system has existed for more than two thousand years. More people are treated with Chinese herbs each year than are treated in any other natural healing tradition. Indeed, Chinese herbal medicines and related methods like acupuncture are used to treat millions of people a year and are available in every major metropolis of this planet.

In the clinical application of Chinese herbology, many natural medicines are used in complex formulas, according to the specific symptom picture of the person. With a complex system of diagnosis, based on a careful listening and examining, the physician determines the specific herbal formula for the individual. Oriental medicine recognizes the interrelation of mind and body and utilizes this understanding in day-to-day treatment. The goal of this healing system is to respect and aid the highly intelligent healing powers of the body by understanding the basic laws of harmony that govern health. Health is understood as balance, wholeness, and vitality. Principles and practice are founded on these fundamental principles of life. This is truly a wise, ecological, and human medical science, which shares fundamental principles with herbal systems, homeopathy, and modern naturopathic medicine. Oriental medicine is blessed with a mature vision of healing that encompasses a rich ecological medical tradition. Not only are these plant medicines clinically effective, they are kind to the body and the earth.

First and foremost, this ecological medicine is based on a principle known as *fu zhen*—the idea that if the body's strength and vigor are maintained, it will not be susceptible to disease. Therefore, there are methods and remedies— based on over two thousand years' worth of clinical experience—to nourish and maintain the great gift of life: energy and health. Exercises like chi kung and tai chi can be practiced to nourish the *chi*, or vital energy, as well as the now common practice of acupuncture. Central to the practice of fu zhen is herbal and dietary medicine. Treatment is directed not toward symptoms or disease labels but to the underlying weaknesses in the terrain of the whole person. Diseases are seen as an expression of different kinds of overall imbalances in the whole person, and in fact each person is treated individually. Current Western medicine has yet to achieve the practical and philosophical maturity of fu zhen, a profound vision of preventative medicine.

Another globally respected system of natural medicine is the Ayurvedic tradition of India. Ayurveda, in existence for thousands of years, is a comprehensive system of health that includes nutrition, herbal medicines, therapeutic bodywork, and spiritual exercises to achieve balance and health. Ayurvedic and Oriental physicians use a good number of the power herbs in this book.

THE ENERGETIC ACTION
OF HERBAL MEDICINES

In the modern era many medical herbalists are trained in the Eastern and Western understanding of herbal medicine. Because Oriental medicine, like Western herbalism, is a vitalistic tradition, it differs from regular medicine in some fundamental principles. Modern medicine considers a person as a conglomeration of chemicals. Chinese medicine sees the body as a living entity; the root of health and life is the *chi*, or vital energy. While the term "vital energy" still raises the hackles of many scientists, from a practical point of view we cannot deny that we are alive and that the combined physical energies of the body could be considered one dynamic whole. Therefore, vital energy need not be a vague or "mystical" concept.

Just as humans are kept alive by vital energy, so too are plants and herbs. Each herbal medicine is a dynamic entity; in other words, it is alive with energy that interfaces with the living human body in different ways. The energetic action of herbs is studied through observation, experience, and intuition. Some of the actions of herbs are easy to understand. Senna, an ancient herbal medicine, helps to move the bowels. One only has to ingest a little bit of senna powder to experience this action! Other herbal actions include sedating the nerves, relieving muscle spasms, and alleviating coughs. All these applications are simple to comprehend. But there is a more complex science of energetics that permeates Oriental medicine.

Understanding the energetic action of an herbal medicine brings one in closer contact to its life and character. Herbs are studied according to their shape, taste, and properties and how these form an energetic character that is unique to the plant. In essence, this energetic character explains how a plant can assist the person when its energy interfaces with the dynamic energy of the body.

Terms like "warming," "cooling," and "nourishing," qualities fundamental to the life in the body, are used to describe the unique characteristics of each herb. For example, American ginseng, one of the premier healing plants of America, is mild and sweet and a moderate stimulant to the overall energy of the body, as well as the lungs and digestive system. It supports the protective energy of the body, what we call the immune system in the West. Clinically, it is prescribed according to a detailed understanding of the person and his or her particular disharmony.

Some herbs, like garlic and ginger, are warming and mildly stimulating, with an affinity for the digestive system; others are cooling—in other words, can moderate the effects of fevers and inflammations. This immensely complex science and art of herbal energetics adds a whole dimension about herbs that is often lacking in dry Western analysis.

The Chinese have been studying and using herbal medicines for centuries, and over the years have compiled valuable books on herbal medicine. These books carefully describe the qualities and properties of hundreds of medicinal substances, based on a comprehensive system of diagnosing "patterns of disharmony," a holistic perspective that is as valuable today as it was in the past. The oldest herbal text is the *Shen Nong Ben Cao Jing;* over two thousand years old, it is attributed to the legendary emperor Shen Nong, who brought much practical wisdom to China.

A more sophisticated herbal, produced by court physicians, appeared during the Tang dynasty around 659 A.D., in an era known for its learning, art, and painting. Medicine also flourished, particularly acupuncture and herbs, led by the incomparable Sun Se Miao, one of the most distinguished physicians of Asian history. His wisdom and medical principles were quite similar to those of the Greek Hippocrates; both shared holistic philosophy and a passion for accurate observation. The most famous herbal in the history of Chinese medicine is the *Ben Cao Gang Mu*, written by the scholar and physician Li Shi Zhen and published in 1596. This monumental volume examines 1,892 remedies, classified in a complex scientific format. Today many of these herbs are found in modern clinics.

In this book I offer a synthesis of the Western and Eastern understanding of the medicinal actions of herbal medicines. Neither is superior to the other, and both are necessary to wholly understand the qualities and actions of medicinal plants.

THE BASIC PRINCIPLES
OF NATURAL MEDICINE

After studying natural medicines for over twenty years, including those of both Asia and Europe, I have seen that all, despite many differences in theory and practice, share basic principles not recognized by conventional medicine. Without understanding these principles, one cannot understand the force and originality of natural medicine. And one could certainly not use the remedies to their best potential. The three major principles are as follows.

First, disease is a reflection of a *disharmony* in the whole body. Diagnosis is aimed at studying the whole and determining the pattern of disharmony so that balance and health can be restored. Bacteria, viruses, and other disease factors are often symptoms of these fundamental underlying imbalances. The whole body/person—what practitioners call the *terrain*—is studied to determine this fundamental underlying imbalance. The study of terrain is the basis of *constitutional healing*, which aims to prevent disease and improve the health of the whole body and person.

Second, all the natural medical systems are based on a *life force*, discussed briefly in the previous section. Treatment is directed toward restoring the strength and harmony of this vital energy. The life force is the basis of all life, of health, and therefore of disease prevention and treatment.

Third, the body contains a healing intelligence, which natural remedies aim to support. While modern drugs can be excellent and necessary, they can overwhelm or harm the body. On the other hand, natural remedies resonate with the body and its energy. They are gentle, nourishing, and effective. Remedies and doctors should aim to support the person and healing intelligence in times of illness and above all *do no harm*.

Ecological medicine is a synthesis of these three principles, an understanding that the human body is a complex integrated ecological system. The main intent is not just to alleviate symptoms but to benefit the whole body and the person and to work with Mother Nature in general, which, I believe, is the aim of all great physicians of whatever background or culture.

In conclusion, it is important to add that in the modern era few practitioners of herbal and natural medicine would discount the advantages of technological medicine and its synthetic drugs. Of course, modern drugs and surgery are important and necessary, but they are only one major segment of the great art and science of healing.

The foundation of all medicine is common sense, positive attitudes, sensible, wholesome diet, balanced lifestyle, and adequate care and exercise for the mind and body. All systems of medicine recognize that most diseases are a reflection of an imbalance in the body, feelings, and mind—the interconnected web of person, community, and nature. Healing, therefore, often calls for more than physical remedies or drugs. It is most often a call for reflection, care, prayer, and the recognition of the web of life of which we are all a part.

PART TWO

HOW TO BUY
AND USE THE
POWER HERBS

WHAT ARE HERBAL MEDICINES?

Herbal medicines are made from plants, often the whole plant, or from a plant's flowers, fruit, root, bark, and leaves, and are most commonly ingested as teas, capsules, and fluid extracts. Herbs can be used in many different ways: in cosmetics, baths, essential oils, homeopathics, ointments, massage oils, and most important for this book, as liquid extracts, tablets, and capsules. Because herbal extracts are a whole medicine with a complex of nutrients and chemicals, they are easier for the body to assimilate than conventional drugs and have far fewer side effects. In the modern age, we are finding out that nature is even wiser than suspected. Research into the constituents of herbs is rapidly proving that nature has provided plants with many compounds that resist disease—properties that inhibit tumors, bacteria, viruses, fungi—as well as life-promoting nutrients and disease-preventing antioxidants.

Vitality and freshness are of great importance in traditional herbal medicine. When an herbal medicine is prepared in a medium of water or alcohol, it imparts chemicals and vitality to the medium. In current Western medicine, the chemicals are thought to be the only source of medicinal power. However, the best herbal companies capture the essence of this life force in their preparations. These remedies, each a remarkable integrated complex of hundreds of constituents, carry their dynamic message into the living human body, healing, nurturing, and reviving.

Traditionally many herbs are prepared as teas, an infusion of herbs in heated water, but some herbs cannot be prepared with this simple process. These require decoction, slowly boiling remedies in water, generally necessary when trying to extract denser plant material like roots and bark. Another time-honored method is to tincture the herbs with a solvent, most commonly alcohol, to extract the medicinal qualities.

Most people do not want to prepare their own herbal remedies. Today many companies manufacture quality herbal medicines, most often in the form of capsules, tablets, and liquid extracts. While I prefer liquid extracts, some high-quality herbal companies also prepare excellent tablets and capsules. Liquid extracts, which hold the potency of the herb very well, do not readily spoil, are easy to use, and can be readily assimilated by the human body. Today, scientific analysis and quality control combine with traditional herbal preparation to create truly fine medicines for modern people.

At home one can prepare herbal teas, a method that is still pertinent in the modern world.

WHOLE HERB EXTRACTS OR
STANDARDIZED EXTRACTS?

Herbal tinctures are prepared from raw herbal material that is soaked (macerated) in a solvent, most often alcohol, which extracts the active healing principles of the plant. Extracts, which can go through several stages of processing, are more complex than a simple tincture and can be more concentrated and purified. Today, the *whole herb extracts* and capsules are subject to complex testing to ensure quality and a range of active constituents, but the preparation of herbs has gone a step further: *standardized herbal extracts*. The standardized preparations, which can be solid or liquid, ensure that what is considered the most active constituent is featured in the final product. For example, St. John's wort is often standardized to 0.3 percent of hypericin.

Many herbal companies now prepare herbs with standardized constituents. Standardization requires several complex stages of extraction, some of which might compromise the whole herb. For example, some companies use toxic solvents like hexane and acetone to "purify" the herb. While the growing tendency to purify and standardize herbs has its good points, the concern is that herbs will become little more than "natural" drugs and an adoption of the pharmaceutical model. It is well known that the integrated constituents of the whole herb extracts are likely to have fewer side effects than the more concentrated preparations.

As long as they do not compromise the whole herb, these new standardized products have their place, but the public needs to be aware that they are buying a more potent herbal product, often best prescribed by a professional. Because the public is susceptible to claims of "potency" and "scientific standards," they often believe these new standardized herbs are better. Many traditional herbalists, Western and Eastern, seriously question this assumption. For example, herbalist Michael Tierra, trained in Eastern and Western herbalism, states that standardization doesn't necessarily make an herb more potent or effective.[3] Furthermore, the public should understand that the "old-fashioned" whole herb extracts are also subject to modern testing and quality control, ensuring a product that is both therapeutic and dependable. The whole herb extracts, or full spectrum extracts, can be subjected to analysis that determines adequate levels of essential constituents.

There is also an ongoing controversy about what is the most active constituent of an herb. An example is the popular St. John's wort, which is often standardized to contain 0.3 percent hypericin, until recently believed to be the most active constituent responsible for the plant's mood-lifting properties. Recently, another constituent, hyperflorin, is said to be as important as hypericin. It turns out the perception of the most active constituent is not as clear-cut as many experts lead us to believe. Herbal medicines can contain hundreds of constituents, all of which can work synergistically to produce the therapeutic benefit, and not all experts agree on which of these compounds are the most active. Many herbalists stand firm on this issue: the health benefits of herbs derive from the synergism of the whole range of chemical constituents. People will ask which is better, the whole herb extract or the standardized extract. Both have their use and

3. *Herbs for Health* 4, no. 3 (July/August 1999): 6.

value, but many traditional herbalists agree that whole herb extracts and teas are, in the end, better for home use.

WHY ALCOHOL?

People often wonder why tinctures and extracts are made with alcohol. Alcohol, which has been used in herbal medicines for hundreds of years, best extracts the medicinal qualities and acts as a preservative. If one ingests a 1-ounce bottle of tincture in a week, the amount of alcohol is minute. However, placing drops of the tincture into a cup of steaming water can evaporate the alcohol, and today, *alcohol-free extracts* are commercially available. Another alternative is to buy the capsules.

HERBAL CAPSULES AND TABLETS

Herbal capsules are quite common on the market and are often preferred to liquid extracts because of convenience and taste. Herbs are simply ground into powder and placed into capsules. There is minimal processing and relatively low cost, but often the quality of the herb is uncertain, particularly for those delicate herbs that lose potency on powdering. The shelf life of capsules is less than that of extracts, and they are more difficult for the body to assimilate. They can come in different sizes, so the consumer must follow instructions on the container, but several capsules are ingested daily, often for up to a week or more, depending on the need or recommendations.

Tablets are herbal matter powdered and crunched, using

tremendous pressure, into a tablet. To make a tablet, additives—excipients like fillers and binders—are included, a process that can detract from the vitality of the herbal remedy. A few companies now make tablets and capsules from liquid extracted herbs and raw herbal material—these are highly recommended. Furthermore, standardized capsules and tablets have recently become available.

TEAS AND INFUSIONS

Teas and infusions are the time-honored, traditional way of ingesting many herbal remedies. Because the boiling of leaves or flowers is generally not recommended, the dried or fresh herbs are placed in freshly boiled water. Tea bags can be used or loose herbs, most often the flowers or leafy parts of the plant. When making herbal teas for healing purposes, people often make them too weak. Place a tea bag (or even two) in a cup of freshly boiled water and steep for up to ten minutes, covered. This produces a strong therapeutic tea, into which lemon, sugar, or honey may be added for taste.

If using bulk herbs purchased at a health food store or herbal pharmacy, place 1 to 2 teaspoons of dried herb directly into a cup or tea ball. Double the amount if you are using fresh herbs. Bring the water to a boil and immediately pour into the cup and let it sit (steep) for up to 10 minutes. Larger quantities can be prepared and stored in the refrigerator to be taken out and drunk at room temperature or gently warmed. Stored herbal teas must be covered well and discarded after three days. If using bulk herbs the final tea must be strained.

Some herbal medicines cannot be made using the tea

(infusion) method. Roots, for example, require gentle boiling (decoction) to extract their active constituents.

Decoctions are water extracts made from the root, bark, berries, or seeds of a plant. Ginseng root, for example, cannot be prepared by the standard infusion method; it must be decocted in water. Break or cut into pieces 1 tablespoon of dried herb and place in a pan, preferably glass, ceramic, or enameled. Pour 2 cups of cold water over the herb, bring to a boil, and *simmer* for 10 to 20 minutes. Do not overboil. Strain. For larger quantities, double or triple the amounts. Drink warm or at room temperature. For some fibrous or tough plant parts, the simmering can go on for up to an hour.

OTHER HERBAL PREPARATIONS

For those people who want to make their own herbal tinctures, the process is quite simple. Generally, I recommend that people buy the many excellent tinctures and extracts on the market; if you want to make your own, consult a book that clearly explains the process. Homemade herbs, when done with care and knowledge, are excellent.

Ointments and oils. Herbal medicines can take the form of *oils, salves, ointments,* and *lotions,* with a variety of important external applications, most notably massage oils and ointments for cuts, muscle pain, and rashes.

Compresses and poultices. Compresses are applied externally for coughs, pains, aches, and other problems. To make a hot compress, also called a fomentation, soak a soft cotton or linen cloth in a hot infusion or decoction. Wring the cloth, as long it is not too hot, and place it on the needy area. As the compress cools, repeat the process. To retain heat and prevent leaking of liquid, put the hot compress in a plastic bag. For inflamed joints, recent sprains, and strains, a cold compress can be made. Headaches often respond well to a cool compress.

A *poultice*, used for pain, poor circulation, and coughs, is an herbal compress made from chopped or crushed fresh herbs.

Essential oils are not herbal extracts but are manufactured in a complex distillation process, producing the essential aromatic oil of a plant with potent therapeutic properties. These highly concentrated oils are only used externally. Often only a drop or two is applied; they can sting or irritate if used around the lips, eyes, and other sensitive areas. People with sensitive skin must not apply pure essential oils directly to the skin and instead should use diluted oils. For sensitive skin, a patch test is recommended; place one drop of oil on a Band-Aid and place on skin for 24 hours. It is well known that the aromas of essential oils have different healing properties, affecting the body, emotions, and mind. Lavender oil, for example, can relax the nervous system. *Aromatherapy*, a distinct branch of herbal healing using essential oils, is a sophisticated healing art with an ancient history. For the home, essential oils can be used three basic ways:

1. to simply breathe in the aroma
2. in a bath, 5 to 8 drops—be sure to stir the water well
3. in massage oils

For massage or other uses, often a drop or two is added to a carrier oil—for example, sesame, soy, avocado, or olive oil. Essential oils have multiple healing potential. For example, they heal the skin, improve breathing, and positively influence emotions. Several superb essential oils are mentioned in this book. Because they are so concentrated, they must be stored out of reach of children.

Baths are a good way to experience the value of herbal medicines in this busy modern world. They are highly relaxing, good for the nerves and muscles, and can have individual therapeutic properties, depending on the herbs used. Herbal bath salts or essential oils are added to a warm bath. Another way to enjoy a bath is to place around 4 ounces of dried herb in a cloth bag and place it directly in the hot bath water. Eucalyptus, chamomile, rosemary, and lavender are some of the best herbs for the bath.

Homeopathic remedies: for a brief overview of homeopathy, see the introduction. Many homeopathic remedies are prepared from common medicinal plants, but homeopathy is not herbal medicine. It is a different but related discipline. Homeopathic remedies are prepared as highly diluted plant essences. Most often they are pellets that are taken in the mouth, often 4 to 6 at a time, repeated 3 to 4 times a day or as directed. These remedies, which come in different dilutions and energetic potencies, are natural medicines that are both safe and effective. Paradoxically, the more diluted remedies have the higher, more active potencies. In other words, 30c, diluted 30 times, is more potent than 6c. The most common potencies for the layperson are 6c, 12c, or 30c or, as is sometimes seen, 6x, 12x, or 30x. If using homeopathic remedies internally, it is best to take them by themselves, because herbs may antidote their effectiveness. Because homeopathy is a complex science and art, only a handful of homeopathic remedies are recommended in this book.

CAN I BE SURE THAT THE PRODUCT I
PURCHASE IS GOOD QUALITY?

This is a legitimate concern for the consumer. It is best to carefully read labels and compare different products. You should look for disclosure of freshness and ingredients and no excipients, additives, or artificial coloring—just the herbs and only the herbs.

With the increasing popularity of herbal medicines, many companies are jumping into the business of selling them. Herbal manufacturing methods can be compromised. For example, some herbs must be prepared from the freshly harvested herb; some companies cut corners and prepare the extract from the dried herbal matter. It also makes a difference when an herb is harvested, how it is handled, and, as I explained earlier, how it is prepared into an extract. However, in America there are now several companies that make good-quality herbal medicines using a fine combination of traditional and modern methods.

The label on the herbal bottle will generally tell the type, source, and quantity of the herb(s). If, for example, the herb has been organically grown, this will be stated. Often the bottle of a liquid extract will have numbers like 1:2 or 1:4 next to the herb listed as an ingredient. These numbers indicate the strength ratio of herbs to alcohol solution. For example, a 1:2 ratio indicates that the extract was made macerating 1 ounce of herb in 2 ounces of liquid. A 1:5 ratio is the internationally accepted standard for an herbal extract. The amount of alcohol can vary from 25 to 95 percent, depending on the needs of the particular herb, but the average is 50 to 60 percent. The label will also indicate the recommended doses and the level of active constituents.

I urge you to ask questions, to shop around, and to not necessarily go for the bargains. The quality of herbal medicines can vary from company to company. Many traditional herbalists prefer the herbal companies that respect the plants and the earth in which they are grown.

What are organic herbal medicines? These are herbal medicines made from herbs that have not been grown in or sprayed with chemicals. The better companies in Europe and America ensure quality control with their herbal medicines and buy them from reputable sources.

Today, I find the best place to buy herbs is the local natural-foods store. Superb natural-medicine pharmacies are now becoming more common, and these are highly recommended.

SINGLE HERBS AND SYNERGISTIC FORMULAS

Herbal medicines can consist of single herbs or combinations. Which is better? Both have their uses and advantages. Some remedies, like hawthorn, are often taken alone; others, like dandelion, are found in superb synergistic formulas. For the busy modern person who has little time to study herbology, a good solution is to purchase a handful of the standard formulas and a few single herbs.

Formulas of herbs contain a mixture of herbs that are known to work well together—they are *synergistic.* In this book I often refer to *synergistic herbal formulas.* They can be excellent medicines. The choice of the several herbs in the formula is the result of much experience and thought. Commercially, there are many formulas for simple health problems: coughs, colds, muscle spasms, bladder irritation, and so on. Both Eastern and Western herbalism extensively use herbal formulas that are reliable for basic health problems. Most current Western research focuses on single herbs, whereas the whole territory of synergistic formulas is largely unexplored. Oriental herbal medicine concentrates on complex formulas derived over generations of experience, while Western herbalists value both single and combination herbs.

ACTIONS AND FUNCTIONS OF HERBS

In the clinic, herbal medicines are understood according to their actions, energetics, and functions. Some herbs are antispasmodic, others relax the nerves (nervines) or move the bowels. There are so many actions and functions of herbs that the subject is too complex for a home guide. In the discussion of each power herb the reader will gain a good understanding of the use of each herbal remedy without worrying about complex terminology that he or she has not been trained to understand.

Most of the fifty power herbs fall into three basic categories: first-aid remedies, detoxifiers, and tonics. First-aid herbs include those that are used for simple problems encountered at home: sprains, cuts, mild headaches and fevers, coughs, and flu. Detoxifiers are traditionally called blood purifiers, a term that indicates that the herb promotes detoxification, neutralizes free radicals and harmful microbes, and promotes the health of the liver, intestines, and whole body. In herbal medicine, detoxifying herbs are an important category because they help the body to rid itself of toxins and wastes and thus maintain the balance of health.

Herbal tonic is a somewhat of an old-fashioned term in the modern world, but basically it is simple and understandable. Herbal tonics nourish and support the organs and functions of the body. Herbalists now prefer such terms as *adaptogen*— an herb that supports the whole body without any harm. Another important category of tonic herbs are those that boost the immune system, a function that is shared by a number of the power herbs.

Some of the power herbs have specific medicinal functions, but for serious health problems these are best left to the professional. It is not recommended, for example, that someone treat themselves for high blood pressure with herbs without professional consultation.

The modern American cannot escape learning some basic terminology about medicinal plants. The field of research into herbs has virtually exploded in the past decade. Several important discoveries have emerged from this research into the constituents that make up plants. Several kinds of plant chemicals have been found to have previously unknown healing qualities.

Some of the key constituents:

> *Carotenoids:* in red, yellow, and green herbs and vegetables; are antioxidants, which protect the body from potentially toxic free radicals.
>
> *Flavonoids:* common in tea, fruits, vegetables, citrus, and many herbs; are therapeutic antioxidants that inhibit carcinogens and heal damaged tissue.
>
> *Indoles:* in greens like kale and cabbage, block cancer-causing substances.

Saponins: in herbs, garlic, and other vegetables; inhibit tumor promoters and improve circulation.

Terpenes: in many herbs and citrus; protect the body from degeneration and disease.

Many of these plant constituents are potent *antioxidants* (a term that is becoming increasingly common). During cellular work the body produces wastes, free radicals, that invade the bloodstream somewhat like terrorists. Antioxidants neutralize these harmful free radicals. It is believed that free radicals are involved in many disease processes, particularly those marked by degeneration and aging. The power herbs contain many beneficial constituents, including vitamins, minerals, and antioxidants.

HOW DO I TAKE MY EXTRACT?

Herbalists believe that the medicinal action of an herb starts right in the mouth with the taste. The bitter taste of a few herbs is part of their healing action! Generally, however, many herbal extracts are quite pleasant and easy to ingest. Most herbal extracts are stored in an opaque dropper bottle. After shaking, drop the recommended dose, anywhere from 5 to 30 drops, in half a cup of water or juice, and drink. It is advised that you take herbal remedies at least one half hour after eating. If taking capsules or tablets, follow the recommendation on the label, but a typical dose is 1 capsule 3 times a day for a few days or more.

For how long? The majority of herbs are ingested for the short term—for example, three times daily for one day or up to a week—and often it is not appropriate to take these remedies for any longer. These would include herbs ingested for first aid, colds, flu, or stomach problems. For example, for a cold, a ginger tea could be drunk 3 times daily for 3 days. Other herbs are ingested for longer, anywhere up to 3 months or even longer, but often with professional guidance. Those taken safely for several weeks or longer are what one might call health promoters, good for rejuvenation, overall health, and prevention of specific diseases. Generally, these tonics or adaptogens work better if used for 2 or 3 weeks, stopped for a period, and possibly used again.

This book, other sources, and the labels offer directions for using these different herbs, but it is important to recognize that for serious or questionable health problems professional guidance is necessary. Most people do not know how to diagnose correctly and have no training in herbal prescribing. Another potential problem is that some people feel that if a little is good, then a lot is much better. Moderation and good sense are necessary if one wants to benefit from herbal remedies.

Dosage. For the home, follow instructions in this book and on labels, but be flexible. Sometimes a small amount of one herb is a lot for one person, a little for another. A large, hefty football player needs twice as much herbal extract as a 110-pound woman. Furthermore, some people are responsive to small amounts of herbs. The amounts recommended on most herbal products are estimated for a 150-pound male. Generally, the doses of herbs do not have to be specific like medical drugs, and if one is asked to take 20 drops but instead ingests 25, there is no need to worry.

Doses can vary according to size, sex, age, body type, and gravity of the health problem. For children below twelve, utilize minimum doses, and seek professional counsel in infants and children under two years of age. Children between six and twelve should take generally less than half of the adult dose. But a robust, stocky twelve-year-old boy can require a different dose from that of a slender, delicate girl of the same age. The elderly generally require about half the dose of an active twenty-five-year-old.

Many herbs should not be used indiscriminately (of course) or continuously over a long period of time, more than two or three weeks, without professional counsel. There are a few herbs, however, that have to be used for a long term to really begin to work, and some, like green tea, can be a part of our daily diet. A few herbs on the market could be toxic when taken in excess, but this is not true of any of the power herbs unless they are grossly abused. Even if herbs are safer than prescription drugs, it does not mean that caution and good sense should be abandoned. For example, herbs like ephedra can be easily abused, and some herbs must be avoided by nursing or pregnant women.

Despite the occasional marketing hype, there are no magic herbs or vitamins for any disease. Disease conditions like arthritis generally require comprehensive care, medical exams and tests, and changes in diet and lifestyle.

HOW CAN I FIND
A GOOD HERBALIST?

In Germany, England, and many other countries this would be a much easier question to answer. In those countries herbal medicine is respected and adequately regulated. In America, few doctors have even basic knowledge about herbal medicines. Furthermore, herbalists, a heterogeneous group, are not monitored, examined, or regulated. But this does not mean that good herbalists do not exist. In rural, ethnic, and urban communities, excellent herbalists can be found via word of mouth. A good herbalist will have a solid reputation in his or her community, will take time to listen to the patient, and will not market herbs or other products. The American Herbalist Guild can be contacted for names of recommended herbalists. Naturopathic physicians often have a good knowledge of herbal medicine. Acupuncturists and herbalists trained in Chinese herbs are knowledgeable about Oriental herbal medicines. A positive recent trend is that a few medical schools are now offering introductory courses in herbal medicine. See the list of resources in the appendix.

PART THREE

THE FIFTY
POWER HERBS

FORMAT

I n this guide each herb is discussed from a historical, botanical, and therapeutic point of view. Scientific explanations,
while important, have been kept concise. The standard references for each herb include the *Complete German
Commission E Monographs*, the *Physicians' Desk Reference for
Herbal Medicines*, and others listed in the bibliography. The
therapeutic perspective includes modern research, as well as
traditional data as understood by herbalists, both Eastern and
Western.

The practical application of power herbs is divided into
three sections: first aid, primary uses, and health promotion.
First aid is self-explanatory. The section labeled *primary uses*
lists those uses recognized by many modern herbalists, but it
is important to understand that in a clinical setting the

medical herbalist concurrently prescribes other herbs or modalities such as nutrition. This section provides information for the layperson to use in conjunction with the health professional. The *health promotion* section describes how power herbs can promote health and well-being. Most of the health-promoting herbs can be taken for a long period, but sometimes only with breaks or with the guidance of a professional. Generally, if one is using a health-promoting herb every day for three months, it is best to stop taking it for a while or seek professional guidance. Most long-term herbs function better when taken for a limited time.

Some entries contain two more sections: *cautions* and *complementary remedies. Cautions* appear if an herb should not be used by nursing or pregnant women or should be used only for a short duration. Pregnant women, for example, must not ingest herbs that stimulate uterine contractions. The heading *complementary remedies* lists those that function well with the herb under discussion or that enhance its therapeutic value.

The basis of natural and holistic medicine is a healthy terrain and a robust constitution. Do not overuse or abuse these remedies, consult a professional when you must, and be humble in the face of the great mystery of disease and health. Often healing comes from places we don't expect and might involve patching up a family relationship or changing careers rather than a drug or natural remedy or could involve antibiotics and surgery or might be best served by prayer and meditation.

FOUR BASIC FACTS TO REMEMBER
ABOUT USING HERBS AT HOME

1. Do not self-prescribe in serious or chronic disease. Consult your doctor in these cases or if you plan to use an herbal remedy for a medicinal purpose while taking a prescription drug.
2. Most herbal medicines are moderate and mild with few or no side effects, but occasionally someone will experience a reaction after using one—most often a rash, a headache, or a stomachache. Discontinue use and, if necessary, consult a physician, but be aware that for the most part these rare reactions go away within a couple of hours. Read carefully about herbal medicines before ingesting them, and know specific restrictions—for example, on use by pregnant and nursing women.
3. If a minor problem does not respond to natural treatment in a week, consult a licensed practitioner.
4. Do not neglect a healthy diet, exercise, and good relationships. There is more to healing than medicines, whether they are natural or synthetic.

ARNICA
Arnica montana

MOUNTAIN MEDICINE

Fitting that arnica should be the first remedy in this book. It is truly premier, a grand solar remedy. The bright, cheerful arnica flowers, which so love the sun, decorate the slopes of mountains and have been used as an herbal remedy in Europe for hundreds of years, especially in the mountainous Alps, where arnica has been used for strains and bruises sustained on the steep slopes and trails. Indeed, one of the common names of arnica is *fall-kraut*—a plant for those who fall. Many American Indian tribes have also valued arnica, which also grows in America. Arnica is applied externally as an ointment, oil, or compress for bruises, sprains, and muscular soreness, and though it has a durable reputation as a wound healer, nowadays it is not applied to cuts or wounds.

Modern herbal medicine values arnica as a massage oil, as a muscle and bruise healer, and to relieve muscular aches. Ignored by regular medicine, arnica was listed in the *U.S. Pharmacopeia*, a compendium of drugs, until 1960. The *Reader's Digest Magic and Medicine of Plants* (1986) states that arnica's only value today is in the garden, a view shared by most conventional books that mention arnica in the past fifty years. A pity, this misunderstanding: arnica is one of the great first-aid remedies of this planet, a valuable remedy for children, athletes, the elderly, pets—in fact, everyone!

Health Benefits. The great German writer Goethe was said to have a great respect for the medicinal arnica, as well as the founder of homeopathy, Samuel Hahnemann. In the nineteenth century Sebastian Kneipp, a famous "nature" doctor, was especially fond of arnica and once prescribed it as a gargle to an opera singer who had lost her voice. Daily gargling with arnica soon got the gratified star back on stage, and to this day we know that arnica can help in this condition: overexertion of the vocal cords. Margery Blackie, physician to the British royal family at the beginning of this century, was well aware of the value of arnica for children who fall, bruise themselves, and cry. No doubt Prince Charles experienced the value of arnica as a boy. In modern times Dr. Rudolf Weiss, a prominent German authority on the clinical use of herbal medicines, calls arnica "a long-established medicinal plant which has been given new interest on the basis of recent research."[4] In the first American herbal physicians' desk reference, published in 1998, once more arnica returns, valued for all its traditional uses.

First Aid. Arnica is a major home remedy for bruises, sprains, strains, muscle *aches* and fatigue from overexertion, shock from accident or trauma, as well as aches and pains from sporting events, labor, gardening, and hiking.

Health Promotion. Arnica homeopathic pellets can be used by families, athletes, and the elderly as a health-promoting herb.

Dose. Herbal arnica is only applied externally, but never on open cuts or wounds because it can create a rash. It is used as a salve, ointment, or compress for the conditions listed. Internal use of the herbal arnica tincture is restricted to professionals. The average person, however, can take arnica internally in its homeopathic preparation: arnica 6c or 12c, taken several times a day for a few days. These are favorably used along with the external treatment.

Caution. External use only—see *Dose.*

---

4. Rudolf Fritz Weiss, *Herbal Medicine*, trans. A. R. Meuss (Beaconsfield, England: Beaconsfield Publishers Ltd., 1991), p. 169.

ASTRAGALUS
Astragalus membranaceus
Huang-qi
milk vetch root

IMMUNE HEALER

One of the major herbs in Oriental medicine, astragalus ranks with ginseng and dong quai and is used daily around our planet in millions of herbal formulas. Its hundreds of years of use have now been verified by modern science. This adaptogen and tonic helps to prevent and cure a wide range of diseases because it supports the protective energy of the body—it stimulates the immune system. Because of its broad efficacy and safety, astragalus now ranks as one of the premier power herbs.

In China astragalus is called *huang qi. Huang* means yellow, after the color of the root interior, and *qi* signifies leader, because this plant is one of the superior tonic medicines. More than 2,000 years ago, astragalus's premier status was recognized in the classic medical text the *Shen Nong Ben Cao Jing,* and since that time it has been found in every major Chinese *materia medica.*

In North America there are nearly four hundred species of astragalus, some of which are poisonous. The infamous locoweeds, which can be toxic to livestock, of the Wild West are a species of astragalus. The therapeutic astragalus is cultivated in China. By the fourth or fifth year of growth, the root is harvested in autumn and dried in the sun, sorted according to size and quality, then cut into thin slices.

Health Benefits. In the Orient astragalus is one of the primary herbs of fu zhen therapy, which aims to balance and support the basic energy and functions of the body and is at the very heart of Chinese medicine. Astragalus, like ginseng, invigorates the vital energy and strengthens the body's defenses. In China it is used along with other herbs to support cancer patients going through radiation and chemotherapy, but it is most often used in formulas with other herbs for colds, weak resistance, and digestive problems. This herb also has some diuretic properties, used to treat swelling and to promote tissue regeneration. Astragalus contains an essential oil, saponins, flavonoids, polysaccharides, and a wide range of fiber, minerals, and vitamins. Scientific research has demonstrated that this herb supports the T-cell function. T-cells, also called killer cells, are components of the immune system that attack harmful invaders. Astragalus is a safe herb that can be taken for quite a long time.

Primary Uses. Promotes endurance, stimulates appetite, and alleviates fatigue; *immune tonic;* for spontaneous sweating, frequent colds, and shortness of breath. It is excellent for the athlete and highly recommended for people recovering from debilitating diseases, overwork, or trauma; also for patients recovering from chemotherapy and radiation.

Health Promotion. Astragalus is a major candidate for health maintenance and promotion.

Doses. Extract, typical dose: 20 to 30 drops 3 times daily up to several weeks, or capsules, often with 300 milligrams of astragalus, 2 to 3 capsules daily. At home astragalus root can prepared as a decoction (9 to 15 grams of crude herb per day), but in Asia it is combined with complementary herbs. Astragalus, found in superb synergistic formulas, is now quite common in America. In combination, American ginseng and astragalus are good for overall energy and for boosting the immune system. Astragalus is an ingredient in a superb tonic for longevity: ginseng, dong quai, and he shou wu in equal proportions (simmered for an hour). If one is purchasing the roots, select the larger roots, up to 3 to 4 inches long: straight, thin slices with yellowish core.

Cautions. Used judiciously, astragalus is a safe herbal medicine.

Note. A chapter on astragalus can be found in *Herbal Emissaries* by Steven Foster and Yue Chongxi.

BARBERRY
Berberis vulgaris

GARDEN SHRUB, GLOBAL REMEDY

Barberry, a deciduous spiny bush, is a common ornamental shrub in America, originally imported from Europe. Many people admire its small scarlet berries, as well as the holly-like leaves and tiny yellow flowers that adorn it during springtime. During the autumn, the leaves' color transforms into a striking pastel pink and orange. In the kitchen, the berries are converted into jellies and jams, but the medicine is prepared from the bark and root.

Barberry has a rich and fascinating heritage. The Egyptians recognized its healing properties and, among other uses, added it to formulas to inhibit the plague—a good idea, considering that it has antibacterial properties. Ayurvedic and Arabic doctors valued barberry, as did many generations of European herbalists and country healers. American Indians were quick to adopt this plant. In *Quincey's Pharmacopoeia* of 1742, an English work, barberry is recommended for diarrhea and dysentery, for jaundice and other distempers from foulness and obstructions of the viscera, and as an ingredient in medicated ales. Dr. Felter, the nineteenth-century American Eclectic, prescribed this remedy for the same problems for which it is now used. Not surprisingly, barberry was one ingredient of the infamous Hoxsey anticancer formula of the 1940s. The controversial Harry Hoxsey, considered a quack by the American Medical Association (AMA), was driven out of business after starting cancer treatment centers. Now we know that several of his herbal ingredients, including barberry, contain antitumor properties—which is not to say, however, that his formula could cure cancer.

Health Benefits. Like many great medicinal plants, barberry is a versatile healer, centered on its affinity for the kidney, liver, digestive tract, most particularly in arthritis and kidney problems. Barberry contains bitter alkaloids that are largely responsible for its antibacterial and antifungal properties, as well as abundant minerals, antioxidants, and vitamin B factors. Modern research has proven that barberry stimulates the immune system and possibly inhibits formation of cancerous tumors. Currently herbalists in Europe and America value barberry as an important blood purifier and a healer for the bladder, kidneys, and liver/gallbladder, but more research is necessary to fully understand this neglected plant. Similar species are valued in Asia for medicinal purposes.

Primary Uses. Herbalists use barberry as a potent blood cleanser, for kidney stones, low back pain, gallstones, arthritis with painful swelling of joints, as well as sore throat, burning urination, itchy skin, inflamed eyes, heel pain, and eczema.

Doses. Extract, tablets, capsules, recommended doses, and synergistic formulas—short-term use.

Complementary Remedies. Oregon grape root is a very similar remedy. Barberry should not be confused with bayberry, a different and useful plant medicine, or with bearberry, another power herb.

Caution. Barberry must not be used for medical problems like kidney stones without consultation with a physician. Avoid during pregnancy unless prescribed by a professional.

BEARBERRY
Arctostaphylos uva ursi

HUMBLE HEALER

Bearberry, or uva ursi, is a humble creeping plant that is common in eastern forests. It is, however, also a global remedy found in North America, Europe, and Asia. A well-known bladder remedy, bearberry has been used by Europeans, Americans, and Asians for many centuries. This small trailing evergreen shrub produces a bright red or pink fruit; it is also called upland cranberry. It often creates a green carpet on open areas in sandy pine forest floors, and its fruit can remain on the plant all winter, providing a survival food for animals and birds. Bears are tremendously fond of nibbling on the little berries, perhaps because they too recognize the healing qualities of the plant. *Uva ursi* means bear grape.

Bearberry has an ancient medical history. Galen, the esteemed Roman physician, used the leaves to treat wounds and stop bleeding. American Indians dried the leaves and mixed them with tobacco, a smoking mixture the Algonquians called kinnikinnik. The nineteenth-century American herbalists were very much aware of the healing properties of bearberry, as were the homeopaths. This plant has an affinity for the bladder; it is used for bladder irritations and infections. A notable astringent, it has a mild diuretic action, but most of its healing benefit stems from its antiseptic properties.

Science has verified the ancient traditional uses of bearberry. Arbutin, the compound largely responsible for the antiseptic qualities of the plant, was isolated from the leaves. Bearberry, however, contains other constituents that have therapeutic actions: flavonoids, allantoin, and volatile oils. Therefore, the whole leaf is preferable to an isolated constituent, as with so many herbs. In *Herbs of Choice,* Dr. Varro Tyler calls bearberry "the most effective antibacterial herb for urinary tract infections."

First Aid. Campers' remedy; for cuts and scrapes the leaves are rubbed on the affected area.

Primary Uses. Bladder irritation or potential bladder infections; kidney stones and prostatitis. Bearberry is one of a handful of useful drainage remedies, those that target a specific organ and clean it. For bearberry to work to optimum, the urine should be alkaline; in other words, avoid acidic foods like citrus fruits and vitamin C while taking this herb.

Doses. Capsules and extracts; recommended dose is 3 times a day for up to 10 days. Bearberry is often used with other bladder/kidney herbs such as horsetail, bucchu, and juniper.

Cautions. Contraindicated during lactation and pregnancy. Short-term use only. Those with heart or kidney problems should consult a professional before taking this herb.

Complementary Remedies. Goldenrod, bucchu, and horsetail.

BILBERRY
Vaccinium myrtillus

MAGICAL PHYTOCHEMICALS

Bilberry, or European blueberry, is another ancient European herb that has been rediscovered in modern times. Bilberry is related to other shrubs that bear delicious berries, including cranberry, blueberry, and huckleberry. Not too long ago this humble medicinal plant was mainly regarded as the source of a delectable fruit—unless you were a student of European herbalism—but because of recent research, bilberry is rapidly becoming a power herb. Indians, country herbalists, gypsies, Shakers, midwives, and many other people have valued bilberry as a food and medicine: to treat scurvy, urinary complaints, diarrhea, diabetes, and dysentery. It has an ancient history; the esteemed Dioscorides, the Greek physician, showered praise on this plant. Within the complex biochemistry of each plant, secrets are being uncovered that reveal that even the most common vegetables contain therapeutic constituents. Bilberry and many of its relatives, including blueberry, black currant, and grapes, contain purple-colored flavonoids called anthocyanosides, bitter compounds responsible for some of the medicinal properties of these fruits.

Health Benefits. Recently it has been discovered that flavonoids have valuable healing properties. There is a confusing array of flavonoids, and the research is ongoing, but it is known that they are antioxidants and that they enhance the effect of vitamin C and strengthen the vascular system. And if that is not enough, it is now suggested they have anti-tumor effects and reduce inflammations. A few intrepid researchers also claim that they work better than aspirin in preventing heart attacks. The flavonoids in bilberry, the anthocyanosides, are particularly numerous, and if that were not enough, this fruit is rich in vitamins and minerals. Bilberry also contains tannins, accounting for its astringent properties and its use for diarrhea and mild inflammations.

All healing plants have stories related to them, some that one must take with a grain of salt. Bilberry is no exception, but here we see one fable becoming fact. Bilberry has a durable tradition of improving night vision. For example, it is said that during World War II the famed British Royal Air Force had a secret weapon—bilberry—that accounted, at least in part, for their success in the nighttime dogfights. The fighters garnished their toast with a much-loved English jam, bilberry. This colorful story is not as far-fetched as it sounds.

Bilberry's flavonoids are said to strengthen and open the capillaries, those tiny blood vessels that penetrate all tissues of the body, including the eyes. Bilberry strengthens capillary walls and prevents capillary leakage. Anthocyanosides, abundant in bilberry, are potent antioxidants, which neutralize free radicals that damage cells.

In Europe bilberry is gaining a reputation because it is said to improve night vision and to reduce eyestrain for many television and computer watchers and seems to be beneficial for the overall health of the eye. Anthocyanosides increase the enzymatic activity of the retina, enhancing the complex chemical conversions in the eye during vision, both day and night. Bilberry is a useful nutrient for those suffering from myopia, retinopathy, cataracts, varicose veins, and easy bruising, and seems to be an excellent herb for all people, particularly the elderly. Although more research is needed to clarify the actions of bilberry, prominent herbalists now recommend it for vision and circulation problems.

Major Uses. Herbalists use bilberry, often in synergistic formulas, to tone the blood vessels, for cold hands and feet, diabetes, dysentery, hemorrhoids, night blindness, varicose veins, and urinary problems. For vision, the standardized extracts are often recommended. The German Commission E, while recognizing bilberry's astringent properties, has not yet approved bilberry for vision problems.

Health Promotion. Bilberry has definitive health-promoting qualities, and is an excellent remedy for elderly people, in fact people of all ages.

Doses. Extract or capsules as recommended, most often twice daily, for several weeks or more. Standardized extracts provide 25 percent anthocyanosides, the recommended portion. Bilberry tea is a good way to benefit from this herb.

Complementary Remedies. Ginkgo and eyebright (power herbs), as well as horse chestnut (*Aesculus hippocastanum*), a remedy used internally and externally for hemorrhoids and other circulatory problems.

Cautions. In recommended amounts bilberry is a safe and nutritive herb.

BLACK COHOSH
Cimicifuga racemosa

INDIAN MEDICINE

Eastern American Indians have valued black cohosh for centuries. One of their names for this plant, squawroot, indicates that it is a plant for women, a use that has been substantiated by modern research. This herb was quickly adopted by white Americans settlers and passed into herbal medicine and homeopathy. Ignored by conventional medicine, black cohosh is still a popular natural remedy, in fact one of the major power herbs for women. Currently this valuable American remedy is making a vigorous comeback.

In the wild, the plant is a beautiful sight to come across. The forest herb grows five to eight feet high, marked by a long delicate plume of white flowers, a source of the name fairy candle. Another nickname is bugbane, because of the odoriferous flowers that can act as an insect repellent. However, the most significant portion of this plant is the hard, knotty rootstock. The name *cohosh* comes from an Algonquian word meaning "rough," a reference to the crusty root.

Health Benefits. Indians favor this plant for menstrual cramping, to alleviate the pains of childbirth, to prevent miscarriage and joint pains, and for insect and snake bites. Modern studies reveal that black cohosh contains anti-inflammatory properties, hence its efficacy in joint and uterine pains. Europeans did not know black cohosh until the nineteenth century when American herbalists—the Eclectics—introduced it to Germany and England. In 1844, Dr. John King introduced black cohosh into Eclectic medicine. A prominent homeopath, Dr. William Boericke, also recommended black cohosh for its broad healing powers, especially for female complaints. A similar plant, *sheng ma*, has been used in Oriental herbalism for many centuries. Sheng ma, valued for pain, infections, and inflammations, is also a cough remedy.

Black cohosh was one of the prime ingredients of several of the most popular patent medicines of the nineteenth century and probably the most effective ingredient of the famous Lydia Pinkham vegetable compound. Naturally, most doctors considered Miss Pinkham's female remedy quackery, but the therapeutic value of black cohosh has now been verified. Still, in 1996 the Food and Drug Administration (FDA) claimed that this herb has no therapeutic value and even warned of potential dangers when using it. Today the German Commission E recommends this great American medicinal plant for menopause and menstrual irregularities.

Primary Uses. Black cohosh circulates the energy and relaxes the muscles and nerves. It is calming, reduces spasms, and benefits the uterus. Herbalists commonly use the herb for premenstrual syndrome (PMS), overstrained muscles, rheumatism and arthritis, nervousness and excitement, changeable emotions, and depression and sadness, particularly when combined with menstrual complaints. Black cohosh is valued by itself and in synergistic formulas for menopausal symptoms. Black and blue cohosh are important female herbs, often used to ease labor pains.

Health Promotion. Notable qualities for health promotion, but generally not for long-term use, unless prescribed.

Dose. Extract, 10 to 30 drops 2 to 3 times daily, or as directed, or one capsule 3 times daily. This herb is found in several excellent synergistic formulas. For menopausal symptoms it is recommended for up to 3 months, then stopped for a period of time.

Caution. Pregnant and lactating women should avoid this herb. Ingested for too long, this herb could cause digestive symptoms, even headaches.

Complementary Remedies. Dong quai, vitex, blue cohosh, and black haw. Black haw (*Viburnum prunifolium*), another Indian remedy, is valued for uterine pains and cramping. Blue cohosh is a gentle tonic for women, especially for uterine problems.

Note. A superb black cohosh review by Steve Foster is in *Herbalgram* 45 (Winter 1999).

BONESET
Eupatorium perfoliatum

COLONIAL MEDICINE

Boneset is another great American medicine that has been neglected in modern times. Herbalists, curanderos, Eclectics, homeopaths, Indians, Southern blacks, and country healers have valued this herb for centuries. Few plants are so American as boneset, as it thrives in damp areas in many eastern states, and has been used by so many different kinds of Americans for so long. A tall, handsome plant, sometimes up to six feet tall, boneset produces pretty clumps of white flowers. Its primary clinical use is for fevers and flu when the patient feels cold to the bones—once called break-bone fever. This bitter-tasting plant is a diaphoretic, that is, it induces sweating.

Early American pioneers and settlers learned of the medicinal properties of boneset from the Indians, who valued it for colds, fevers, and flu. Virgil J. Vogel reports that many tribes, including the Iroquois and Mohegans, favored boneset. In 1852 Dr. Clapp reported to the AMA that boneset

5. Virgil J. Vogel, *American Indian Medicine* (Norman, OK: University of Oklahoma Press, 1970).

6. Ibid.

"deservedly holds a high rank among our indigenous medical plants."[5] During that time boneset became extraordinarily popular; its dried flowers were found hanging in most barns, and it was drunk hot "during the cold stage of fever," as reported by the Confederate Dr. Porcher.[6] So popular was boneset in the nineteenth century that it was elevated to a panacea, an unfortunate development because it obscured its true value. We forget, however, what life was like in the era before central heating, good plumbing, and antibiotics. Houses and villages were often damp and cold, and people were more susceptible to colds, muscle aches, and flu. Boneset and willow bark (which contains constituents that became aspirin) were the aspirin of those times.

Herbal critics have often lambasted poor boneset, another herbal quackery they claim, but in Germany, where herbal medicine is treated with respect, boneset is valued for its immune-enhancing properties and it is confidently recommended for colds and influenza. Boneset also has mild anti-inflammatory properties and has some value in arthritis. Research also makes the intriguing suggestion that this humble plant might shrink tumors. One of the key constituents of boneset, sesquiterpene lactones, are being studied for their immune-enhancing and antitumor potential.

Primary Uses. Colds, flu, and fevers, especially when the patient feels cold and shivers; acute bronchitis, fevers, coughs, and arthritis.

Doses. Capsules and extracts, suggested doses. Warm sweetened tea from flowering tops is a good use of this bitter-tasting herb, 2 to 3 times daily. Boneset is a short-term herb.

Complementary Remedies. Peppermint, elderflower, and yarrow.

Caution. Avoid boneset during lactation and pregnancy. The homeopathic preparation can be used.

BURDOCK
Arctium lappa

WILD FOOD, POTENT MEDICINE

One of my favorite wild foods, which is also good when cultivated, is the tenacious burdock. Not well known to Americans, except as a persistent weed with sticky burrs, burdock is appreciated by Japanese and other Asians for its earthy taste, nutrition, and medicinal qualities. In Japan it is called *gobo.* Burdock, a biennial weed, is stout and bushy and spreads itself with the tenacious burrs. Second-year burdock, harvested in late summer or fall, is preferable for food or medicine. By the end of summer, the plant produces small globular purple flowers on stems as high as six feet.

Like most weeds, fecund burdock loves to spread itself wherever it can take root and is especially common in damp vacant lots, along fields, and on the edges of farms. However, burdock can be cultivated, as it is in Asia, and along with other more common vegetables like carrots, spinach, and kale, it makes a hearty addition to our diet. In Asian dietetics, burdock root is valued as a tonic. Resembling a long brown carrot, it is a yang, robust food that strengthens the body. It is good for the tired, weak, or convalescent, and as a gentle tonic for active men and women. Folk medicine sometimes calls it an aphrodisiac; for that, alas, I could not find any evidence.

Shakespeare, who was familiar with many plants, mentions burdock in several of his plays. For example, in *Troilus and Cressida*, Pandarus says, "They are Burs, I can tell you, they'll stick where they are thrown." Because of the infamous burrs, this plant acquired several colorful nicknames, including *clot-bur* and *beggar's buttons*. Like yarrow and St. John's wort, this wonderful weed thrives over much of our planet and is found in all major medical traditions except modern American medicine, which steadfastly claims that burdock is simply a weed. Quite recently, an "herbal expert" blandly claimed that no evidence exists that burdock has any "useful therapeutic activities." Here again the pharmaceutical companies have not rushed into burdock research, but recent studies discovered that the fresh root contains polyacetylenes, compounds with antibiotic and antitumor properties.[7] Clearly, this plant has medicinal properties.

Burdock has long been a favorite of European and American botanical physicians. The famous medieval German abbess Hildegard of Bingen was a healer well versed in the medicinal use of European natural medicines. She was one of many to use burdock to treat growths and swellings. Aspiring Indian medicine men were said to fast for a week, only drinking burdock broth to clear and strengthen the body and mind. Russian herbalists have long considered burdock a potent

7. Kazuyoshi Morita, Tsuneo Kada, and Mitsuo Namiki, "A Desmutagenic Factor Isolated from Burdock (Articum Lappa Linne)," *Mutation Research* 129 (1984): 25–31.

healer. Burdock has a long history of use in formulas that assist those suffering from cancer and other chronic diseases.

Health Benefits. Burdock root has been appreciated as a food and medicine by many American Indian tribes and generations of European herbalists. The Eclectics in America favored this potent root and called it a powerful cleanser of the blood, kidney, liver, and lymph glands. The whole plant can be used to prepare medicines, including the leaves, flowers, and seeds, but the root is the most common medicinal part. The root contains bitter glycosides, flavonoids, alkaloids, tannins, a trace of oil, inulin, resin, and mucilage. In Chinese medicine burdock seeds are commonly used to heal septic conditions like boils and abscesses and especially for sore throats. In Western herbalism, the root is praised for its use with skin problems and arthritis. With other herbs, burdock is prescribed for eczema, psoriasis, and boils and is found in formulas that help cancer patients. No evidence exists that burdock alone can cure cancer, but research has discovered that this common weed has diuretic, antibacterial, antifungal, and antitumor properties. A superweed—certainly similar in its potential to two other power herbs, nettle and St. John's wort—burdock is quite clearly a neglected medicine.

Primary Uses. Traditionally burdock has been used as a "blood purifier," to cleanse the liver, kidney, and digestive tract and for arthritis, stones, and skin inflammations. Externally, it is applied to red irritating skin problems. For specific health problems, burdock is best prescribed by a professional.

Health Promotion. Burdock has some deep healing properties but it is generally used for a limited period of time. The fresh root, a nutritious food, can be a part of our diet and seems to be the best source of the medicine, at least for its tonic properties. In the West the specific medicine is often made from the dried root.

Doses. Extract or capsules, recommended doses, as well as preparations of the fresh root. Burdock extract is a safe herb, but for the average person it is best used in synergistic formulas for the short term. A decoction can be prepared from a heaping teaspoon of the root in 3 cups of water. Drink several times daily.

Caution. Pregnant and lactating women should consult a physician before using this herb.

Complementary Remedies. Red clover, dandelion, and yellow dock.

CALENDULA
Calendula officinalis
Marigold

FLOWER REMEDY FOR FIRST AID

The marigold is a much-loved flower and natural medicine, most respected in Europe, where it has been used for centuries. The pale green leaves and golden-orange flowers are a lovely addition to any garden. The botanical name, *Calendula*, comes from Roman times, when it was said that the plant bloomed on the first day or "calends" of every month. Like all common European herbs, the marigold has been mentioned in countless stories and poems. Particularly interesting to poets is the fact that the flower expands and closes with the sun, creating the poetic image of the awakening of the "weeping flower." In *The Winter's Tale*

Shakespeare refers to "the Marigold that goes to bed wi' the sun / And with him rises." The medieval *Grete Herball* says that "maidens make garlands of it when they go to feasts or bridals because it hath fair yellow flowers and ruddy."

However, there is more to marigold than beauty. This plant is a power herb of ancient lineage, its history going back to the Greeks and Egyptians. Amazingly enough, this remedy turns out to be global; Asians and American Indians also value it. Traditionally, marigold was also found in the kitchen, added to soups, salads, conserves, and candies. The medieval monks and herbalists raised calendula in their medicinal gardens. Charles Stevens, in *Maison Rustique, or Countrie Farme* (1699), says that marigold is a specific for headaches, jaundice, red eyes, toothache, and ague, and that farmers use the flower tea to strengthen the heart. During the Civil War, marigold was made into an ointment to slow bleeding. The nineteenth-century homeopaths adopted this famous natural medicine, using it in their hospital wards and first-aid kits.

Health Benefits. Today calendula is immensely popular in soaps, shampoos, and cosmetics, as well as medicinal lotions and ointments. The medicine is prepared from the flowers and leaves. This soothing and gentle healer is perhaps the major remedy for the skin, particularly abrasions, chapped skin, minor cuts, and rashes. It is a major first-aid remedy in homeopathy and modern herbalism. Traditionally, calendula has been used to slow bleeding and for the healing of wounds and skin ulcers. It is also used internally for digestive inflammations, ulcers, and gallbladder problems. In herbalism calendula is known as a blood purifier and as such is used for inflammations like measles, chicken pox, and fevers.

Calendula, a premier home remedy, is good for the whole family. It can even help babies, diaper rash, and dry skin. It has antifungal properties and can retard the growth of pernicious bacteria, and it is often used to heal simple cuts and abrasions. Calendula tincture on a cotton ball washes cuts and chapped skin. A calendula lotion or ointment can be applied to scars, and the soap is a superb cleanser and deodorizer. Calendula tea can be used as a mouthwash and gargle.

First Aid. Abrasions, sores, wind chafing of the skin, cuts, itching, minor burns, ulcers, bruises, varicose veins, and hemorrhoids.

Primary Uses. Herbalists use this herb internally for menstrual cramping, gastritis, eczema, ulcers, fevers, and digestive disorders.

Health Promotion. Historically, calendula has been used for skin and other cancers, though no modern research supports this use yet.

Doses. Calendula is available in tinctures, oils, lotions, teas, creams, and ointments. Calendula ointment is a good foundation of every home medicine kit. An excellent tea can be made from calendula flowers to be used as a lotion, beverage, or compress.

Caution. Internal use with caution for pregnant women.

Complementary Remedies. Externally for the skin: aloe vera, calendula, St. John's wort, comfrey, and tea tree oil. Aloe vera is best used from the fresh plant leaf.

CHAMOMILE
Matricaria recutita

THE SUN GOD

The Germans, who have appreciated chamomile for many centuries, still add this most famous herbal remedy to teas, medicinal formulas, and cosmetics. Early Teutonic tribes dedicated the herb to the sun god because the flower, with about eighteen white ray florets around a yellow conical center, resembles the sun. The flower heads, rich in phytochemicals, are the most therapeutic part of the plant. There are two major kinds of chamomile, Roman and German, which are almost identical from a medicinal point of view.

A power herb of great distinction, ancient lineage, and versatility, chamomile ranks with St. John's wort, garlic, and echinacea as one of the superstars of natural medicine. A great harmonizing herb, chamomile has been appreciated in most healing traditions. The Greek Dioscorides, one of the great herbalists of the ancient world, respected chamomile, as did the Ayurvedic physicians of India. Perhaps no other medicinal herb has been so commonly used in Europe since ancient times. Nicholas Culpeper, the London herbalist of the seventeenth century, gave the good advice of bathing in chamomile to "remove weariness." Not only is chamomile deeply relaxing but also it is healthy for the skin. In Europe, the value of chamomile is legendary. Even Peter Rabbit was served chamomile tea to soothe his upset stomach. In *The Tale of Peter Rabbit* Peter eats himself sick in Mr. McGregor's garden and is then chased out by the irate gardener. What is a good rabbit to do? Peter goes home, where his mum serves him a hot cup of chamomile tea.

In nineteenth-century America when clinical herbalism thrived under the Eclectic physicians, chamomile was often recommended. Besides the universal uses, Dr. Felter valued the medicine for wounds, menstrual cramping, children's colic, and diarrhea. Like the homeopaths, the Eclectics recognized that therapeutic chamomile had, like most medicinal plants, a value in alleviating emotional states, in this case for those who are irritable, fretful, and impatient. No wonder this plant remains such a popular remedy.

Health Benefits. Primarily known as a pleasant apple-scented beverage in America, chamomile is regarded by many herbalists as far more than a folksy home remedy. Dr. Rudolf Weiss says that in recent years the reputation of chamomile has changed drastically: "Recent pharmacological and clinical studies show chamomile to be a very important medicament, an example of what can happen when plants long established in popular medicine are made the subject of proper scientific study."[8]

The major effects of chamomile are due to its volatile oils; therefore, it is important to use the fresh herb for remedy preparation. The volatile oils, including azulenes, have several proven health benefits, but the plant also contains flavonoids, coumarins, polysaccharides, and numerous vitamins and minerals. Studies have demonstrated that chamomile is indeed valuable for indigestion because it relaxes the smooth muscle lining of the digestive tract. This power herb may also prevent stomach ulcers. It is a major remedy for the whole digestive tract and a premier medicine for children and women. It relaxes the nervous systems of all people. Because

8. Weiss, *Herbal Medicine,* p. 24.

it is a mild antispasmodic, it relaxes the uterine muscles and therefore can be used for menstrual cramping. This power herb also stimulates the immune system, a valued action for colds and flu. The nineteenth-century Eclectics were right on when they prescribed the use of chamomile externally for cuts and wounds. It reduces inflammations, stimulates the cells to heal, and inhibits harmful bacteria. Chamomile is an easy herb to grow, and it is quite durable, so much so that it (the Roman variety) even thrives when it is stepped on! A power herb indeed.

First Aid. External use for cuts, abrasions, and dry, irritated skin. A strong tea for relaxing effects.

Primary Uses. Herbalists use this herb alone and in synergistic formulas for many conditions, including ulcers, emotional tension, restlessness, headaches, coughs, painful menstruation, sluggish digestion, bronchitis, gallstones, inflammations, arthritis, and dermatitis. Homeopaths use this herb for cross and irritable patients who are fussy, changeable, and demanding. This is an excellent remedy for children.

Doses. The most common use of chamomile is the tea. Extracts and capsules are also excellent. For external use there are compresses, lotions, and creams. Chamomile is an important cosmetic herb. For a bath, use 5 drops of the essential oil, or tie a handful of flowers into a cloth and put into the bath. These baths are highly recommended for fatigue, stress, and colds. Chamomile is found in countless herbal formulas because of its harmonizing and versatile healing qualities.

Dr. Rudolf Weiss, one of Europe's experts on the clinical use of herbal medicines, gives the following formula for coughing. The treatment is to inhale the vapors of the steaming herbs. A handful of the chamomile flowers are placed in a bowl, hot water is poured over them, and the patient breathes the vapors while wearing a large towel over the head and the bowl. Thyme might also be added to this most wonderful remedy.

A hot strong cup of chamomile tea—sometimes mixed with linden and elder flowers—makes an excellent tonic to sweat off a fever and flu.

Cautions. Very occasionally someone might be allergic to this very safe herb, which, by the way, can be ingested by pregnant and nursing women.

DANDELION
Taraxacum officinale

THE TEETH OF THE LION

A pity that in Western culture dandelion has been labeled a useless weed and that its therapeutic powers are all but ignored, and how ironic that this prolific plant is doused with poisonous herbicides in lawns across our land. This humble "weed" is just the kind of medicine that many Americans need.

Dandelion, like many great medicinal plants, is seemingly indestructible, as it flourishes in yards, back lots, and anywhere it can set its roots. *Dent de lion*, the Old French name for dandelion, refers to its sharp serrated leaves: the teeth of a lion. The cheerful dandelion is a handsome little plant. Its yellow flowers brighten many lawns and meadows. The whole plant, root and leaves, is a highly nutritious vegetable that is still appreciated in Italy and other countries where it is cultivated or picked in the wild. Dandelion is a universal healing plant, like yarrow and St. John's wort—hardy and versatile medicines that grow all over the world. A favorite of country folk, herbalists, midwives, and even poets, dandelion has graced our lawns, gardens, and meadows for thousands of years. "Shockheaded Dandelion / that drank the fire of the sun."—Robert Bridges

In the old days dandelion had a list of colorful common names, including *swine's snout*, *priest's crown*, and *piss-a-beds*. The genus name of the plant, *Taraxacum*, is a reflection of its healing powers: in Greek, *taraxos* means disorder, and *akos*, remedy. The Arab physicians of the tenth and eleventh centuries were the first to write about dandelion in the West, calling it *taraxacon*. Clearly, dandelion's special properties were widely recognized in former times. Nicholas Culpeper, the British herbalist, put dandelion under the dominion of Jupiter, the expansive planet known for its healing powers. In the body dandelion opens and cleanses, particularly the spleen, liver, and kidneys. Culpeper explains: "You see here what virtues this common herb hath, and that is the reason the French and Dutch so often eat them in spring; and now if you look a little farther, you may plainly see without a pair of spectacles, that foreign physicians are not so selfish as ours are, but more communicative of the virtues of plants to people."[9]

Incredibly enough, dandelion is used by herbal traditions all over the world, including American Indians, Arabs, Chinese, and Europeans, but it is not recognized in any way by conventional medicine. After all, it is not only a mere plant

9. Nicholas Culpeper, *Culpeper's Complete Herbal* (London: W. Foulsham, 1952).

but also a common weed! Dandelion contains no high-powered alkaloids that can be extracted at vast expense, and it will never make millions of dollars for a pharmaceutical company, but in its totality it is a valuable and versatile healer.

Dandelion was once listed as a medicine in America but, like most herbs, was abandoned at the beginning of this century. The Eclectic doctors of the last century commonly used extract of fresh dandelion for jaundice, skin disorders, rheumatism, and gastritis. Some herbalists even consider the wild dandelion a better source of medicine than the cultivated plant. Research has demonstrated that the active bitter principles in dandelion are more abundant in the wild root.

Dandelion is a nutritious plant with an extraordinary balance of major minerals. Traditional herbalism considers dandelion a blood purifier, that is, it treats a broad terrain disharmony that signifies dysfunction of the liver and impurities in the lymph and blood, resulting in skin problems, headaches, swollen glands, and irritability, and mood changes. In China dandelion is added to complex herbal formulas for breast and other cancers, though no evidence exists that this remedy can cure cancer. The fresh leaves have diuretic properties.

Primary Uses. Modern herbalists prescribe dandelion for a wide array of problems, often in combination with complementary herbs: arthritis, gout, skin eruptions, gallstones, liver diseases, and high blood cholesterol. It also is nutritive for nursing mothers and convalescents.

Health Promotion. One of the great inexpensive remedies for health promotion and longevity, dandelion restores vibrancy and health to the blood and slows degenerative conditions when used with adjunct remedies.

Doses. Decoction and extract made from the root; extract, 10 to 30 drops several times per day, as recommended; also capsules and tablets. The dandelion greens are a highly nutritious food; one cup has more vitamin A than one carrot.

Caution. Those with gallstones should consult an herbalist when using this herb. There are no known contraindications for pregnant or nursing women.

Complementary Remedies. Red clover, milk thistle, blessed thistle, burdock, and sarsaparilla.

Note. The FDA claims that dandelion is a weed with no therapeutic properties. They should have read Ralph Waldo Emerson: "What is a weed? A plant whose virtues have not yet been discovered."

DONG QUAI
Angelica sinensis

MOTHER OF HERBS

Dong quai, a major Oriental herb, is found in many herbal formulas. While it is the main "women's" remedy in Oriental medicine, dong quai is used to excellent purpose in many "male" formulas. This herb, prepared from a large root, is also one of the best-selling traditional medicines outside of China; it is included in many formulas, teas, extracts, pills, tablets, and even shampoos.

Dong quai is the major blood tonic in Oriental medicine. The Oriental meaning for *blood* in medicine is broader than the Western meaning. While blood is the fluid running through our blood vessels, it is also considered a yin energy that nourishes and supports the yang, or active, energy of the body. Blood tonics are extremely important for both women and men, because we all exist in a changing flux of yin and yang.

One of the several meanings of *dong quai* is "to return to order." Because Oriental cultures recognize the central role that women play in the family and culture, they give great importance to herbs that improve the health of women. A nutrient-rich herb, dong quai is loaded with minerals and vitamins that support the human body, including vitamin E and iron. This herb, however, is rarely used alone in Chinese herbalism; most often it is combined with synergistic herbs in countless formulas for a wide range of health problems. Modern research has discovered that dong quai has several constituents that positively affect the liver, blood, uterus, and nervous system. Rich in nutrients like iron and cobalt (a constituent of B_{12}), this herb contains a rich profile of key compounds, including terpenes, oils, astringents, and bitter saponins. Dong quai is said to nourish the blood, promote circulation, regulate menstruation, nourish dryness, and move the intestines. For centuries Oriental women have used this herb for beauty, for vigor, and as an overall tonic. It is said to soften the skin when taken internally.

Primary Uses. An important herb by itself but best used in formulas to enhance absorption. Valued for dry skin, lack of or abnormal menstruation, painful menses, anemia, uterine bleeding, constipation due to dryness, chronic pelvic problems, abdominal pain, traumatic injuries, fatigue from stress and overwork. It is commonly found in formulas to improve one's sex life, for infertility, as well as in many formulas for children, men, and the elderly.

Health Promotion. A fundamental herbal tonic.

Doses. Extracts, capsules, and synergistic formulas. Can also be prepared as a decoction. Like astragalus, the roots are whitish and sliced into slivers. The larger the root and the sweeter the flavor, the better the quality. It can be eaten raw after a very light steaming (cut into thin slices). It has a unique celerylike flavor and is often added to soups and stews.

This herb is a major ingredient in the famous *Shou Wu Chih*, a popular tonic for overall energy and health. Another simple preparation for a gentle tonic: take 2 cups of water and 1 root sliver and cook with half a cup of schisandra berries. Simmer until 1 cup remains. Drink half a cup in the morning, the rest in the evening for a week or so. A nourishing chicken soup can be enhanced by a few slices of dong quai, particularly for those who are tired, pale, and weak.

Found in many formulas, dong quai enhances the action of other important herbs like ginseng and astragalus. A decoction or extract combined with astragalus is excellent for fatigue, warmth, and circulation in winter. An essential herb for menstrual difficulties, especially pallor, excessive blood loss, fatigue, irritability, tinnitus, and blurred vision.

Complementary Remedies. Black cohosh, red raspberry, astragalus, ginseng, vitex, schisandra, saw palmetto, and blue cohosh.

Cautions. Avoid during diarrhea or heavy uterine bleeding. Dong quai is not recommended for lactating or pregnant women (except under the guidance of an Oriental herbalist) or for those on blood thinners.

ECHINACEA
Echinacea angustifolia
Purple coneflower

PURPLE CONEFLOWER

Purple coneflower, so named because of its distinct and handsome flower, is one of the great American herbal medicines. Once broad fields of echinacea could be admired in many parts of the Midwestern prairie, but nowadays its natural habitat has shrunk because of farming and development. The purple flower has become a very popular decorative plant and can now be found all over America. Ironically, many gardeners grow this perennial without realizing that it is a major medicinal plant. Echinacea (*E. purpurea*) can be readily purchased at most garden stores, and once planted in a sunny location it returns each year, spreading gradually. It blooms in the summer for many weeks, a tall, handsome plant crowned by a handful of the distinct purple flowers. Few plants have such durable flowers, thus accounting for its popularity in modern gardens. It needs minimal care. The medicine is made from the whole plant, but the root is the most important part.

All the Midwestern tribes prized the coneflower, most notably the Sioux nation. Among other things, Indians used the remedy for snake bites and wounds. The dried flower, with its symmetrical spikes, was also used as a comb by the Plains Indians. One pioneer, Edwin Denig, who became friends with the Assiniboin people who lived along the Missouri River, reported that this flower was their most important medicine.

It is called by the French *racine noir,* and grows everywhere in the prairie throughout Indian country. It is chewed and applied in a raw state with a bandage to the part affected. We can bear witness to the efficacy of this root in the cure of the bite of a rattlesnake or in alleviating pain and reducing the tension and inflammation of frozen parts, gunshot wounds, etc. . . . Its virtues are known to all the tribes with which we are acquainted, and it is often used with success.[10]

Before the era of antibiotics, echinacea was a great gift because of its immune-enhancing, antibiotic, and antiviral properties. Echinacea was heartily adopted by early white settlers and hunters, then absorbed into botanical and homeopathic medicine. It was a major remedy of the Eclectic physicians of the last century. At the beginning of this century, conventional medicine declared that echinacea had little medicinal value. When the Eclectics were legislated out of business in the 1920s, echinacea was just about forgotten—until the Germans began testing it in the mid-1900s. Once the bane of conventional doctors, echinacea has made a resounding comeback, a testament to the genius of John King, John Uri Lloyd, and Harvey W. Felter, the great herbal physicians of the late nineteenth century.

Ironically, this most American of medicines is hardly known by conventional medicine in United States but is enthusiastically used in Europe, where it is one of the best- selling natural

10. Kelly Kindscher, *Medicinal Wild Plants of the Prairie* (Lawrence, KS: University Press of Kansas, 1992), p. 86.

remedies. Echinacea is a major healer, primarily of the immune system, its value supported by hundreds of scientific papers. According to German studies, the actions of this herb are partly due to water-soluble polysaccharides that have immune-stimulating actions and some antimicrobial properties. It is no doubt a useful plant medicine, especially since it is nontoxic.

First Aid. Echinacea is a first-aid remedy for cuts and abrasions.

Primary Uses. Activates the immune system, restrains infections, and clears toxins. Herbalists use it alone and with other herbs for inflammations, fever, swollen glands, sore throats, irritable bladder, and inflamed prostate gland. Externally, it is applied to cuts and boils. The German Commission E approves echinacea "as a supportive therapy for colds and chronic infections of the respiratory tract and lower urinary tract."

Health Promotion. Echinacea is a classic herb for health promotion, but should only be used conservatively. See the restriction under doses.

Doses. Extract, 15 to 30 drops 2 to 3 times daily; also found in capsules or tablets; use as directed. An excellent tea can be brewed from the dried or fresh herb. Versatile echinacea is utilized in compresses, douches, lotions, cosmetics, and synergistic formulas. Like many natural remedies, the best echinacea is prepared from the whole fresh plant, a process neglected by some companies. When one puts a few drops of echinacea (*E. angustifolia*) extract in the mouth, it creates a tingling sensation, a sure sign of a good product. Echinacea purpurea does not create this sensation but is considered equally therapeutic.

Cautions. A safe herb by any standard, but it is best not to take echinacea regularly for more than ten days without a break. Many people take echinacea too frequently. The body will respond better to most natural remedies if they are used correctly. Furthermore, patients with AIDS, cancer, or autoimmune diseases should seek professional counsel before using echinacea.

Complementary Remedies. Goldenseal, baptista, thuja, chaparral, and osha.

ELDERBERRY
Sambucus nigra

THE PEOPLE'S MEDICINE CHEST

Few plants are as versatile as the remarkable elderberry bush. Historically, few have been held in such high esteem. In the modern world, elderberry has been a forgotten medicinal plant—until very recently. Elderberry is a familiar bush and small tree in America and Europe. In England, where it is very common, elderberry marks the coming of summer with its flowers and the immanence of autumn with its ripening purple berries. Maude Grieve, renowned British herbalist, reports many culinary uses of the abundant berries, including for jellies, chutneys, and vinegar. The fragrant umbrella of white flowers is as familiar a sight as the drooping bunches of purple berries. The word *elder* comes from an Anglo-Saxon word *aeld*, fire, because the hollowed-out branches were used for blowing up fires. The botanical name *Sambucus* is said to come from the Greek word *sambuca*, for a stringed instrument, but because of its hollow wood it is more likely that elder was used to create wind instruments.

When I was a boy growing up in New York State, we had a prominent elderberry bush in our garden. The branches, easy to hollow out, could be easily converted into blowguns and whistles. Imagine my delight when I discovered that this was a common practice back in the Middle Ages and Roman times. Pliny, the Roman historian, mentions that boys would make toys and weapons from the elder branches. Furthermore, the wood of the elder has been converted into panpipes and flutes for as long as we have written records.

Elderberry has also been associated with healing and magic and has been used by gypsies and other country folk as a protector against evil. In his *Art of Simpling* (1656) William Cole writes that country folk used elder "to prevent witches from entering their houses." The branches and leaves were hung above the doors and windows. Strangely enough, elder has also been associated with grief and sorrow, and there are legends that claim that Judas hung himself on an elder and that the Cross of Calvary was made from the wood. Elderberry has long been a favorite of witches and country healers, but more important are its considerable healing properties. Its reputation is testified to countless times through the ages. Naturally, Shakespeare was well aware of elder the medicine. In *The Merry Wives of Windsor:* "What says my Aesculapius? my Galen? my heart of Elder?"

Health Benefits. The therapeutic qualities of elderberry have been valued for thousands of years. Indeed, evidence of its use can be found in Switzerland reaching back 10,000 years. Romans, Greeks, gypsies, English country folk, witches,

Italians, Shakers, and many other people have used elderberry as a medicine, a use for which it is extraordinarily versatile. In North America, eastern Indian tribes were well versed in the medicinal qualities of this plant. In the nineteenth century American herbalists and homeopaths were quick to adopt it as a medicine. However, with the advent of modern drugs at the beginning of this century, elderberry, like many great natural medicines, was sorely neglected. However, I am pleased to announce that elderberry has recently had a remarkable resurgence in the world of natural medicine, due to its inherent therapeutic potency and supporting scientific research. Elderberry is now a valued power herb. From Israel to America, elderberry has made a comeback because it is a potent remedy for colds, flus, and coughs, and scientific research has verified that it supports the immune system.

Elderberry is a complex medicinal plant because several parts can be used and each has distinct medicinal uses: the berries, leaves, bark, inner bark, and root. It is no wonder that elderberry has been referred to as a medicine chest. Hippocrates and many others mention the bark as an emetic and diuretic. The berries are commonly made into a tonic wine, and the seeds converted into diverse medicines. The flowers, the very apogee of elder's growth, have been used for cosmetic purposes and to beautify the skin of women, as well as for colds and sinus problems. The leaves have been applied to bruises and sprains and might even have some antitumor properties.

In 1993 a double-blind study in Israel demonstrated that elderberry (*Sambucol*) could relieve the symptoms of flu better than a placebo or a synthetic drug. How could this humble plant have such powers, defying all the dogma against natural medicines in the modern world? Pernicious viruses invade the body like enemy rockets and use spikelike projections to introduce their enzymes through the protective membrane of the healthy cells. Elderberry extract neutralizes this invasion. But this is not all. Elderberries are a rich source of flavonoids that stimulate the immune system, particularly by boosting the production of lymphocytes, "killer cells," a second line of defense against nasty invaders. Furthermore, elderberries contain one of the highest levels of vitamin C in nature, as well as flavonoids like quercetin, a potent antioxidant. This natural remedy is indeed a power herb.

First Aid. Preparations from the leaves are used for sprains, bruises, and minor burns.

Primary Uses. Two different remedies are used: the flower tea for colds, flu, upper respiratory problems, sinusitis, and hayfever. The berry, a gentle stimulant for the immune system, is also valued in flu and mucus-related problems—a good remedy for children.

Health Promotion. Elderberry contains properties that support the immune system and overall health.

Dose. For the flowers or berry extracts, capsules and synergistic formulas are available. The flower tea, which I highly recommend, is prepared like any other tea and used 2 or 3 times a day for a few days. The berry extract, a valuable winter remedy, is found in syrups and tonics.

Notes. For constituents and a synopsis, see *Herbal Medicines,* by Carol A. Newall, Linda A. Anderson, and J. David Phillipson.

ELECAMPANE
Inula helenium

BREATHING RELIEF

Legend has it, according to John Gerard, that the world-famous beauty Helen had a clump of elecampane in her hands when Paris stole her from Menelaus, thus precipitating the infamous Trojan War. It is no surprise that this distinctive plant, a global power herb, should be the source of legends and poems. Also called wild sunflower, elecampane is a tall handsome plant with a sturdy stalk, large green leaves, and cheerful sunny flowers. A hardy perennial, it makes a welcome addition to any garden.

An ancient medicinal herb, this neglected healer deserves a revival in the modern world. It was valued by Greek, Roman, Chinese, Ayurvedic, and European herbalists and was adopted into American herbalism. Primarily a lung and stomach remedy, elecampane is used for coughs, chest colds, digestive problems, and asthma. The Greek physician Dioscorides respected this plant, as did the Romans. Pliny, the Roman historian, tells us that "Julia Augustus let no day pass without eating some of the roots of Enula, considering it to help digestion and cause mirth."[11] In past centuries the plant was candied and chewed for flavor and to ward off "poor humors" and "pestilent airs." Nicholas Culpeper tells us: "The fresh roots of Elecampane preserved with sugar or made into a conserve, or a syrup, are very effectual to warm a cold windy stomach and stitches in the side . . . and to relieve cough, shortness of breath and wheezing in the lungs."[12]

11. Maude Grieves, *A Modern Herbal* (New York: Dover, 1971).

12. Culpeper, *Culpeper's Complete Herbal*.

Health Benefits. Culpeper was right on the mark with elecampane, even appreciating its use in "pestilence"—a use confirmed by scientific research. At the beginning of this century American herbalists, including the Eclectics, used elecampane. In 1922 Dr. Harvey W. Felter, in his Eclectic compendium of medicines, wrote that it "is of great service in bronchial irritation with cough of persistent or teasing character, with copious expectoration." The beneficial effect on the lungs is still recognized by modern herbalists and, indeed, elecampane is a power herb specifically for the lungs, an expectorant found in many cough syrups. It has, however, also been used to treat the stomach, colon, and skin and was a major veterinary medicine for skin problems of horses. It even gained a nickname: horseheal.

The root contains the complex carbohydrate inulin, a starchy material that swells and forms a slippery suspension when mixed with digestive fluids. Burdock and marshmallow roots also contain inulin. The Orientals recognize that this plant is a powerful healer of the lungs and a soothing medicine for lower bowel disorders. In Oriental medicine the lungs and intestines are polar organs that have a strong influence on the skin, a picture that perfectly fits the healing pattern of elecampane. Interesting too is the perennial association of elecampane with happiness and "mirth," emotions that are said to be depleted with weakness in the lungs.

The root also contains a potent essential oil (consisting primarily of sesquiterpene lactones) that can rid intestinal worms and has antifungal, antibiotic properties. The past use of elecampane to rid "pestilence" therefore has some rational basis, as does its potential for healing problems of the colon.

The plant is also rich in nutrients, particularly zinc, thiamin, and magnesium.

Primary Use. Tiredness combined with shortness of breath, unproductive cough, deficient resistance, melancholy and sadness, feeling of wanting to give up and better lying down, chronic bronchitis, lung cold with phlegm, and poor appetite.

Doses. Extract, capsules, and synergistic formulas, standard doses, sometimes 2 to 3 times daily for a week or so. This remedy can also be prepared as powders, teas, salves (for the skin), cough syrups, wines, and candy.

Complementary Remedies. Coltsfoot, hyssop, elderberry, horehound, thyme, and yarrow. Mullein is another remedy for bronchitis, especially when there is a hard cough with soreness. I recommend herbal cough syrups with combinations of these herbs. Highly recommended for the lungs are the durable garden herbs hyssop and thyme, best made into extracts from the fresh flowering plants to capture their remarkable healing essence.

Cautions. Pregnant and nursing women; also diabetics.

EYEBRIGHT
Euphrasia officinalis

GOOD CHEER

Euphrasia, a Greek word that means "good cheer," is a happy name for this elegant little plant, which is decorated with tiny white or lilac flowers. A curious herb, eyebright is semiparasitical in that it needs other plants to survive. Of course, poets have not neglected this lovely little plant. To the English poet John Milton it was known as euphrasine. The great poet relates how the Archangel Michael ministered to Adam after the fall:

> *. . . to nobler sights*
> *Michael from Adam's eyes the film removed,*
> *then purged with euphrasine and rue*
> *His visual orbs, for he had much to see.*[13]

Another durable herbal medicine, eyebright is very much alive in the contemporary world of botanical and homeopathic medicine. As its name clearly indicates, this herb has an affinity for the eyes. The pretty little flowers resemble an eye. The law of signatures, a belief that irritates modern plant scientists, is a traditional belief in folklore: within the shape, form, or color of a plant are clues to its medicinal uses. This holistic view derives from the fact that herbalists traditionally believed that the Creator is the force behind all creation, including medicinal plants, on which the stamp of intelligence can be observed. Of course, there is some nonsense to the applications of this belief, but it does work some of the time. Modern plant researchers, however, have ignored eyebright; it does not yet have the modern scientific blessing like the more popular garlic or echinacea. This astringent herb is, however, official in the *British Herbal Pharmacopoeia* and maintains a durable tradition in herbalism. In fact, eyebright has established its own little niche in natural healing that will just not go away.

Health Benefits. Hildegard of Bingen, one of the most renowned herbalists of the Middle Ages, valued eyebright.

13. Grieve, *A Modern Herbal.*

Nicholas Culpeper has this to say about eyebright: "If the herb was but as much used as it is neglected, it would half spoil the spectacle maker's trade and a man would think that reason should teach people to prefer the preservation of their natural before artificial spectacles, which they may be instructed how to do, take the virtues of Eyebright as followeth."[14] Alas, good Nicholas was much ignored then as now, despite the fact that his writings contain gems of truth. However, he would be glad to know that eyebright has not been deserted by modern herbalists in America and Europe, even if it cannot ruin the trade of spectacle makers. While it is not considered a cure for problems of vision, it is an important remedy for the eyes, sinuses, and head. The great homeopathic physician William Boericke, recommended eyebright for sinusitis, itchy eyes, and excess mucous discharges. David Hoffman, a modern authority on herbs, says that it is an excellent remedy, particularly for colds and sinusitis, as well as inflammations of the eyes with itching and weeping. From the Oriental medical viewpoint one calls this herb cooling and drying, with an affinity for the eyes, nose, lungs, and liver. In Oriental medicine it is said that the health of the eyes is connected to the health of the liver. Remedies that are good for the liver are indirectly good for the eyes. Eyebright is rich in vitamins and minerals, as well as tannins, resin, bitter compounds, and flavonoids. On the whole, eyebright is a rare remedy that is healthy for the liver and the eyes, but it is a plant that needs more research and study.

Primary Uses. Runny nose, flu, hay fever, conjunctivitis, sore throat, red swollen eyes, and stinging and burning eyes.

14. Culpeper, *Culpeper's Complete Herbal.*

For hay fever, it is often combined with stinging nettle, for sinusitis with goldenseal, and with elder flowers for colds, runny noses, and itchy eyes.

Doses. Extract, teas, tablets, and capsules; eyebright is generally taken 2 to 3 times a day for several days to a week or so. Traditionally an eyewash is prepared from the tea, but the German monograph does not recommend this use. Commercial eyewash preparations of this herb are now available. Eyebright is found in excellent synergistic formulas, particularly for sinusitis and hay fever.

Complementary Remedies. Stinging nettle, bilberry, pulsatilla, and elder flower.

FEVERFEW
Chrysanthemum parthenium

HEADACHE RELIEVER

A handsome plant that thrives in gardens with little work on the part of the gardener, feverfew is common in many American gardens. Feverfew, however, is a distinct plant with its own healing powers and, as it name implies, has a reputation for reducing fevers. In actuality the name was *parthenion* (having to do with "girl") in ancient times, changed to *featherfoil*, for its feathery leaves, to *featherfew*, and then *feverfew*. Many people declared that this was a good fever remedy. Others still use it for women's problems. Some have valued the plant for headaches. Feverfew demonstrates the confusion that circles around some herbs until substantial studies are completed.

Traditionally feverfew has a long history, but in the twentieth century it fell into disuse, even among herbalists. In the 1970s, however, the herb came bounding back when some studies verified that it could relieve the most insidious form of headache, the migraine. In fact, feverfew was one of the herbs that marked the beginning of the modern renaissance of herbal and natural healing. In the 1960s, when science began to cast its wise gaze over quaint, old-fashioned herbology, it began to find some remarkable facts, most notably that herbs really do work.

Feverfew has been traditionally used for fevers, arthritis, menstrual pains, and headaches. Culpeper said that feverfew can reduce "all paines in the head."[15] Feverfew, however, remained a relatively obscure remedy and was not much used in America by the nineteenth-century Eclectics, homeopaths, or herbalists. The story changed in England in the late 1970s. A miner recommended a home remedy, feverfew, to the wife of a chief medical officer of Britain's National Coal Board. After trying this curious remedy, the woman experienced relief from her recurrent headaches. Her husband brought the news of this success to a Dr. E. Stewart Johnson, who happened to be in charge of a London migraine clinic. He cautiously tried the remedy on a handful of his patients, found some success, and went on to oversee a major double-blind study of lowly feverfew—one of the first such major studies on an herbal medicine. This study was followed by yet another that confirmed the results of the first. Two large groups of headache patients participated, one receiving feverfew, the other a placebo. Feverfew outperformed the placebo significantly. Feverfew made the headlines and even found its way into one of the most prestigious medical journals, the *Lancet*.

One of the most ancient uses of feverfew, dating back

15. Ibid.

to Dioscorides, is for female problems, most notably menstrual cramping. One ingredient, parthenolide, is anti-inflammatory, validating its use for pain, cramping, arthritis, and fevers. Feverfew is somewhat like the modern aspirin, which is itself derived from an herbal remedy.

First Aid. Headaches; the leaves can be chewed; or extract or capsules can be taken.

Primary Uses. Headaches, migraines, mild fevers, and menstrual cramping.

Doses. Fresh leaves, 2 or 3 times daily; capsules or extract for a week or so, 2 or 3 times daily. For migraine sufferers: take regularly for at least 6 weeks; some recommend standard doses with at least 0.2 percent of parthenolide.

Caution. Avoid during lactation or pregnancy; and minor side effects have been reported, including mouth ulcers and digestive upset. Do not take any medicine for a prolonged time for headaches that do not go away—see a physician. While feverfew can relieve migraines, stubborn headaches can have several causes that need comprehensive examination. In Oriental medicine acupuncture and a variety of herbal formulas are used with some success.

GARLIC
Allium sativum
Da-suan

GLOBAL REMEDY

A universal natural remedy and culinary spice, garlic has been appreciated by the Chinese, Indians, Egyptians, Europeans, and many other peoples for thousands of years. No other medicinal plant, with the possible exception of ginger, has been valued by so many peoples for so long. In modern times this popularity has not diminished. In California alone over 250 million pounds of garlic are harvested each year. Many of the great cooks of the world, most notably Italian and Chinese, make great use of this much-loved plant.

Garlic belongs to the lily family, along with another medicinal food, onion; they are among the oldest cultivated plants known. The first written mention of garlic dates from around 3000 B.C.; garlic's therapeutic benefits are praised on a tablet of Sumerian cuneiform. The world's oldest extant medical text, the Egyptian *Ebers Papyrus*, makes repeated mention of garlic. Egyptian priests placed onion and garlic on the altars of their gods, and several garlic bulbs were found in the tomb of Tutankhamen, placed there more than a thousand years before the birth of Christ. We should not be surprised that this superfood is mentioned in the Bible. When the Israelites fled from Egypt to the promised land, they lamented the lack of good food: "We remember the fish, which we did eat in Egypt freely: the cucumbers and melons and leeks, and the onions and garlic" (Numbers 11:5).

In the ancient world, garlic was fed regularly to slaves and soldiers to keep them healthy, from Egyptian pyramid builders to Roman soldiers. The greatest doctor of ancient Greece, Hippocrates, extolled the virtues of garlic, as did the most eminent physician of Roman times, Dioscorides. Even the world's most famous wanderer, Ulysses, ingested garlic to protect him, not against germs, but against the dreaded sorceress, Circe. In all cultures that give importance to the spirit world, garlic has been valued as a universal guardian, even against the feared vampires. Garlic has been placed over

countless doors to keep out the invisible, unwanted guests—
not the same reason that modern chefs decorate their kitchen
walls with braids of dried bulbs. Garlic was also an ingredient in many antiplague formulas—certainly one that had
genuine germ-inhibiting properties.

During the third century the Romans introduced garlic to
England. Naturally, Shakespeare mentions the clove. In *A
Midsummer Night's Dream*, the comic actor Bottom says:
"And, most dear actors, eat no onions / nor garlic, for we are
to utter sweet breath." To the detriment of the rich, garlic was
often sneered at by the aristocracy, who considered "fetid garlic" a peasant food. This peasant food, the humble garlic
clove, has been used in countless wars as a germicide and to
treat wounds, and even as late as World War I garlic was used
by European physicians. With the discovery of penicillin in
1928, garlic fell into eclipse, but it was still treasured by thousands of Russian soldiers during World War II when their sup-
plies of penicillin ran out. For a time garlic was known as
Russian penicillin.

Health Benefits. Since ancient times many therapeutic
powers have been attributed to garlic, giving it the aura of a
wonder healer. As it turns out, some of this praise is war-
ranted. Garlic is not just a fable of folk healers and sorcerers.
It is a power herb. The Ayurvedic medicine of India has
respected garlic for several millennia. When the British first
went to India they observed that many of the lepers consumed garlic avidly, so much so that "peelgarlic" became a
term for leprosy. A dreaded and insidious infectious disease,
leprosy has been feared since biblical times. Ironically, modern science has validated that garlic can indeed inhibit the
germ that causes leprosy.

Oriental medicine has valued garlic for centuries. The first record of medicinal use is found in Tao Hong-Jing's *Ming Yi Bei Lu (Miscellaneous Records of Famous Physicians)*, published in China around 510 A.D. In China garlic is phenomenally popular with the millions of poor peasants who use it as a disease preventative as well as for illnesses ranging from colds to digestive problems to tuberculosis.

The esteemed French scientist Louis Pasteur first recognized garlic's antibiotic activity in 1858. Since that time his work has been substantiated in hundreds of studies. A primary antibacterial compound in garlic is allicin, which is only released when the garlic bulb is chewed, chopped, or crushed. Garlic is also known to contain antifungal properties, but it is universally respected for its health benefit for the blood and heart. The one obvious setback is the pungent odor and taste. Herbalists agree that garlic is most potent in "the raw," not emasculated or processed. For people who don't want to eat the raw clove, garlic can be generously added to meat and vegetable dishes, and garlic capsules can be purchased for those who want its health benefits without the sting. Put into water, garlic loses some of its therapeutic benefit. In Chinese herbalism garlic is considered a warm and spicy food that promotes vital energy and circulation, kills worms and bacteria, detoxifies, and purifies. Like many great natural remedies, garlic is extremely rich in nutrients, including calcium, phosphorus, sulfur compounds, iron, thiamin, riboflavin, and vitamin C. It also contains antioxidants like germanium and selenium. Garlic is truly a superfood, a supermedicine. Today garlic is universally recognized for its multiple healing properties, and hundreds of scientific papers testify to renewed interest in this most venerable medicinal food.

First Aid. Garlic juice on minor cuts and abrasions, bites, and stings.

Primary Uses. To promote digestion and circulation; to prevent colds, sinus problems, coughs, and viral infections. Also used to treat parasites, pinworms, and bacterial infections. Garlic is often best during cold season, when the amount can be doubled in food or eaten raw. Some other uses include: a drop or two of garlic, diluted with a bland oil, in the ear for infection. Garlic keeps the blood vessels clear, eliminates toxic metals, and supports the immune system. Not surprisingly, garlic is being researched for cancer prevention.

Health Promotion. Clearly garlic is a superb food to consume daily and has many properties to aid in the maintenance of good health and long life.

Doses. Fresh garlic for the brave; or garlic lightly sautéed and then eaten. Garlic extract can be found alone or in synergistic formulas. Processed garlic products should deliver at least 5,000 micrograms of allicin daily.

Complementary Remedies. Propolis, shiitake, reishi, osha, echinacea, ginger, cayenne, olive oil. Onion, garlic's cousin, is also healthy for the heart and blood.

Note. To eliminate garlic breath, chew the traditional breath fresheners: parsley, fenugreek, or fennel. Garlic is easy to cultivate from the cloves, which are broken off the bulb and planted in the ground in the autumn.

Caution. While garlic does have bona fide antibiotic properties, it should not substitute for antibiotics unless directed by a physician. Excess raw garlic—more than four to five raw cloves a day—can be harmful.

GINGER
Zingiber officinale
Chiang

SPICY MEDICINE

Ginger is one of the most common kitchen spices in the world. The zesty ginger root, not too long ago an exotic item in America, is now found in all supermarkets. Throughout the tropical belt of the world, ginger is fabulously popular, consumed by thousands of tons every year, and it is just as popular for its medicinal qualities, which, according to some books, are legion. Ginger, originally from southern Asia, now flourishes in Africa, South America, and the Caribbean. An erect perennial herb 2 to 4 feet tall, it grows from thick white tuberous rhizomes.

Ginger's history is as ancient as any herb, cultivated by Hindus and Chinese for centuries. The esteemed Chinese philosopher Confucius (551–479 B.C.) mentioned ginger in his *Analects,* and it is included in the famous *Ben Cao Gang Mu* of Li Shih Jen, as well as many other Oriental herbal compendiums. The Greek physician Dioscorides makes frequent references to ginger in his *Materia Medica*, describing its warming effect on the stomach and its benefit for digestion. It is even mentioned in the holy book of the Muslims, the *Koran*, as an herb served to the righteous in paradise.

During the European Middle Ages ginger was an important item in the lucrative trade from the East. The tremendous need for ginger and other spices for medicine, preservatives, and spice created fortunes, wars, and vigorous commercial rivalries. Ginger traveled to Europe through Arab nations. The shrewd Arab merchants controlled the trade for many centuries, and because of pirates, poor transportation, exorbitant taxes, and uncertain borders, ginger traveled a rough, uncertain route. The great need for cheaper and more abundant spices—including pepper, cardamom, and ginger—was one of the reasons that Europeans began to look for a new route to the East Indies and India, centers of the spice production in the world. Portuguese, English, French, and Spanish began a vigorous era of exploration and colonization that would change nations, eating habits, and agriculture. The greatest of all explorers, Columbus, was looking for an easier route to the wealthy Spice Islands. On the way he discovered America. It is not far-fetched to say that spices like ginger drastically changed the history of this planet.

By the sixteenth century, ginger was successfully grown on Caribbean islands like Jamaica. Ginger thrives in hot, wet, tropical climates and grows easily and abundantly. In favorable conditions one acre of land can produce more than 1,500 pounds of dried ginger. Naturally, it is an integral part of cooking in most tropical countries.

During the Middle Ages ginger was a popular spice in England, so much so that it entered the English language. In England to ginger something up means to give it life and zest. The English grew extremely fond of ginger in meat dishes, bread, candy, and even beer. It has even been joked that the English started their vast Asian empire to ensure a steady supply of tea and ginger. In Shakespeare's *Love's Labours Lost* Costard informs Moth: "An I had but one penny in the world, thou shoudst have it to buy ginger-bread." Spicy, warming ginger was a perfect antidote to the cold damp weather of the British Isles. Today ginger finds its way into breads, pies, cookies, pickles, syrups, soft drinks, candies, and countless delectable Oriental dishes.

Health Benefits. In the Orient, ginger, revered as a gift from the gods and a versatile medicine, is found in ancient grave sites, temples, and altars. Naturally it also finds its way into most kitchens, from the most humble to the fanciest restaurants in Hong Kong and Beijing. Every Oriental herb pharmacy from Vietnam to America carries this spice. Ginger is an important ingredient in countless Oriental herbal formulas because it allows more potent medicines to be readily assimilated by the body, and its distinct warming qualities perk up digestion, energy, and circulation. Many common problems like colds, muscle aches, and upset stomachs respond well to ginger.

First Aid. Fresh ginger juice can be applied to insect bites and minor burns. Ginger juice mixed with sesame oil is used to massage tired or aching muscles. Externally, ginger compresses and poultices are applied for abdominal cramps, colds, and muscle soreness. One simple application is to take fresh ground ginger, about 1/2 pound, strain the juice through cheesecloth, and rub it into the muscles. For those whose muscles feel worse in damp weather, ginger tea can be drunk and the juice rubbed into the affected muscles.

Major Uses. Motion sickness, morning sickness, and nausea; for colds, particularly damp colds with postnasal drip; muscle aches and pains. Ginger is an aid to digestion, especially when there is gas and belching, and is valued for circulation, headaches, and arthritis.

Doses. Fresh preparations, capsules, and extract. Ginger can be used in cooking for its medicinal effects, but most effective is the ginger tea or extract. Tea is made by squeezing ginger juice into a cup of warm water, by simmering diced ginger, or by adding 15 to 20 drops of extract to a cup of warm water. Synergistic formulas of ginger are available.

Cautions. Those who are sensitive to spices should be sparing with internal use of ginger. For the short term, a pregnant woman can use moderate amounts of ginger, but it is best to seek professional advice.

GINKGO
Ginkgo biloba
Bai-guo

JURASSIC MIND MEDICINE

Thanks to Steven Spielberg, we all know that dinosaurs flourished during the Jurassic period. Incredibly enough, we have a power herb whose relatives also flourished during that remote time; ginkgo, also called maidenhair tree, is now one of the superstars of botanical medicine. In the past decade it has received much publicity on account of scientific studies that have validated its remarkable therapeutic benefits. Ginkgo, considered one of the oldest living tree species on earth, is the only surviving member of the primitive ginkgo family, one that flourished in the days of dinosaurs. The ginkgo tree, the superman of trees, can live more than 1,000 years and is like the legendary phoenix that rose from the flames of destruction. Many instances have been recorded where a ginkgo tree resurrected from ashes in temple or urban fires. A ginkgo tree is even reported to have survived the blast of the atom bomb at Hiroshima.

Englebert Kaempfer, a German surgeon working for the

Dutch East India Company, described ginkgo in 1712. In his notes the name *ginkgo* first appeared, probably an adaptation of the Japanese pronunciation of a Chinese name for the tree. The tree has been cultivated for hundreds of years in the Orient, where it was favored in parks and temples. Recently ginkgo has been imported into the West, where it is in common use along urban streets owing to its resistance to air pollution and disease. It is a lovely tree with distinctive fan-shaped leaves, a full, round shape, and thick leafy growth. The fresh seeds of a ginkgo tree are considered toxic, and children should be warned. Once the acrid pulp is removed, the seed is boiled or roasted and is considered a delicacy in China and Japan. Like many great herbal medicines, ginkgo is also the subject of much Oriental poetry and painting.

Health Benefits. In medicine, two parts of the tree are commonly used. In China the seeds, which must be prepared to reduce the mild toxicity, are used to treat asthma and urinary problems and to benefit overall energy. I will focus on the leaves, which are nontoxic; in Oriental medicine they are said to promote blood circulation, alleviate pain, benefit the lungs, and act as a tonic to the brain—to "awaken the brain." Not surprisingly, this quaint description is the truth. Ginkgo has a close affinity for the brain and the thinking processes.

The popular contemporary use of the ginkgo leaves is largely a product of European scientific research. Today in France and Germany this once esoteric tree produces one of the highest-selling natural medicines. Ginkgo is now primarily used for circulatory problems, arteriosclerosis, forgetfulness, and loss of memory. European scientists have conducted over three hundred studies on ginkgo's therapeutic benefits.

It is now said to help Alzheimer's patients. Numerous double-blind tests have confirmed the effectiveness of ginkgo. One German study revealed an astonishing improvement of 72 percent in elderly patients who took the herb for brain disturbances. Another positive Dutch study, published in the *Lancet*, the prestigious British medical journal, validated that ginkgo can improve circulation to the brain and possibly slow dementia and other signs of senility. Scientists have extracted flavone glycosides and ginkgolides, unique substances that they believe are the most active constituents. In brief, ginkgo's health benefits are based on several interrelated actions: it is a potent antioxidant that protects cells from damage; it reduces formation of clotting; and it appears to reduce inflammation and activate the brain cells.

Ginkgo is now known throughout the planet, but it has found its greatest use in Europe. In France ginkgo is so popular that the French have started a huge ginkgo plantation in South Carolina in the United States, a region and climate conducive to good production. Quite recently Americans have begun to discover the benefits of this extraordinary tree. Curious that a tree so famous for its durability should have analogous medicinal qualities. Ginkgo is, without doubt, a power herb.

Primary Uses. To improve circulation, memory, and cognitive functions. Ginkgo has potential for patients who have suffered strokes and could very well prevent strokes. There are indications that this herb can improve hearing and diminish some cases of ringing in the ears (tinnitus). Herbalists also use the leaf extract for those with cold extremities, impotence, asthma, and dizziness. Furthermore, there is evidence that ginkgo can improve flow of blood to the heart and slow the degeneration of sight caused by macular degeneration, the leading cause of adult blindness.

Health Promotion. The potential of ginkgo is tremendous, especially when combined with a wholesome diet, sufficient essential fatty acids, and good vigorous exercise. Ginkgo is less likely to help sedentary people who consume poor-quality fats, smoke, and do not ingest sufficient fresh vegetables. Ginkgo is not for continuous long-term use; see *Caution*.

Doses. Extract, capsules, and tablets, use as directed. Also found in synergistic formulas, particularly with gotu kola, another power herb. Some authorities praise the standardized extracts, ensuring a minimum of active constituents. A typical dose might be 40 milligrams 3 times a day for 2 to 3 months.

Caution. While ginkgo is a health-promoting herb of high standards, it is not recommended that it be used for more than three months without a substantial break. Dizziness, fatigue, and headaches have been reported with long-term use. Those on blood thinners should consult a professional before taking this herb.

Complementary Remedies. Bilberry, gotu kola, and ginseng.

Note. One of many studies about the therapeutic value of ginkgo: Pierre Braquet, "The Ginkgolides: Potent Platelet-activating Factor Antagonists Isolated from *Ginkgo Biloba* L.: Chemistry, Pharmacology and Clinical Applications," *Drugs of the Future* 12 (1987): 643–99.

THREE GINSENGS

ARISTOCRATIC HEALERS

Ginseng, one of the premier herbal medicines of the Orient, is also one of the most famous on this planet. There are several different kinds of ginseng. In this book I focus on the three most commonly used: Chinese, American, and Siberian. In China ginseng is one of the "kingly" remedies of the herbal tradition. It is said that Mao Tse-tung, Chou En-lai, Deng Xiaoping, and the rest of China's aging communist hierarchy—many of whom were quite vigorous even in their eighties—began each of their conferences by passing around a tray of the most select roots. These roots, grown in a special plot in the Manchurian mountains, are still carefully guarded, as they have been for hundreds of years—the special reserve of Chinese leaders of whatever political persuasion. This plot, planted with seeds of the finest wild stock, was taken over by the Communists when Mao triumphed in 1949. Do you think they destroyed this prime vestige of aristocratic privilege?

There are many names for ginseng in China and other cultures. It is called spirit vessel because of the kindly nature of the spirit associated with the plant. Many ancient people believed that the root was a condensation of earth energies vital to humans. In Tibet ginseng is called the medicinal plant giving long life. Other laudatory names can be found in Japan, Korea, and India. Shen Nung, an ancient Chinese herbalist, said of ginseng: "Ginseng is a tonic to the five viscera, quieting the animal spirits, stabilizing the soul, preventing fear, expelling vicious energies, brightening the eyes and improving vision, opening the heart, benefiting the understanding, and taken for some time will invigorate the body and prolong life."[16] This resounding reputation has survived for over two thousand years.

AMERICAN GINSENG
Panax quinquefolius

American ginseng, a superb indigenous natural medicine, grows in the mountains of the East from Vermont down to Georgia. Like its Oriental counterpart, American ginseng grows on a single stem, 6 to 12 inches high, which produces small, serrated leaves. In late summer the plant produces a fruiting stalk and a clump of small green berries that ripen to a bright red. It is unethical to harvest the plant before the berries have fallen. In fact, it is preferable to leave the wild plants alone. Each year the root patiently gathers its essence and strength from the rainwater, the sun, and the rich black loam of decaying hardwood leaves.

Prior to the arrival of the white man, the Atlantic region was a vast virgin forest filled with massive oaks, beech, and other precious hardwoods and conifers. This forest, particularly in the mountains, harbored many medicinal trees, mushrooms, and plants, of which ginseng was one of the aristocrats. Inhabiting much of this region was the proud Iroquois nation, a people intimate with the many uses of all plants and trees. Ginseng, one of their sacred plants, was called man's thighs

16. Ron Teeguarden, *Chinese Tonic Herbs* (Tokyo/New York: Japan Publications, 1984), p. 78.

and legs separated because of its humanlike shape. The Chinese call the plant *Jen-shen*, which means man root. The special affinity that ginseng has for human beings was intuitively recognized by both races.

Not all tribes valued ginseng as much as the Chinese, but some, like the Creeks, used it much as the Orientals did. For example, they favored it for asthma and emphysema and to help warriors regain their strength after being wounded. The Indians also added ginseng to their love potions, those that aroused passion as well as those that would "bag" the game—in other words, make the user irresistible to the object of their desires.

It was a Jesuit priest, Father Petrus Jartroux (1669–1720), who was responsible for introducing American ginseng into the Chinese market. He asked a colleague who was working with the Mohawks near Montreal to mail a sample to another Jesuit in China. The Chinese were impressed with the taste and quality of this related ginseng, and soon they became anxious to import more. Thus began the strange, obscure saga of an American commercial enterprise: a vigorous trade in ginseng that continues to this day. Indians, pioneers, and frontiersmen became "seng" hunters, selling bags of roots to middlemen who would ship them west on riverboats and horses to the port of San Francisco. Though a tiny chapter in American exportation, ginseng trade is not insignificant. Daniel Boone is reputed to have lost a small fortune when his ginseng boat tipped over in the Ohio River.

To meet the growing demand, a small circle of farmers began to cultivate the finicky plant in the nineteenth century. However difficult the plant, there are financial and other rewards in a successful crop. In 1989 over two million pounds of cultivated ginseng, valued at 54 million dollars, was exported to the Orient. Over 200,000 pounds of wild ginseng was exported the same year, at a much higher cost per pound.

It is sad and ironic that the great bulk of this most healing plant is exported to the Orient, while Americans inundate their bodies with toxic chemicals. This paradox is another reflection of a basic fact about health: in Oriental medicine, the prime focus is to preserve the balance of health, particularly the vital force. Ginseng is one of the major healing plants for maintaining the balance and vigor of health.

Today, ginseng is used all over the world, in teas, tablets, syrups, complex formulas, and patent medicines, as well as shampoos and cosmetics. Its reputation has spread beyond the circle of herbalists, acupuncturists, and Orientals. It is a favorite, along with a handful of other special herbs, of professional athletes. Ginseng is now finding its way into the mainstream. Some companies now produce standardized ginseng extracts, expensive little pills of high quality that can be purchased at local pharmacies.

In conventional medicine ginseng has never been appreciated. Even the homeopaths and Eclectics made little use of this plant. In the last century, regular doctors were quick to proclaim ginseng a quack's medicine, an opinion that was never seriously examined. Undoubtedly, one reason for this dismal label was prejudice. What could the Chinaman know? Another hurdle was the bias against medicinal plants; they were deemed ineffective and weak, incapable of the power of chemical drugs. Medical science has been slow to study this plant because it doesn't fight any particular disease. Instead, like other adaptogens, it improves the functioning of the whole body.

To understand the healing properties of this plant, it is important to examine the experience of the Chinese herbalists. American ginseng (*xi yang shen*) has been a major medicinal herb in the Oriental pharmacopoeia for several hundred years. Its Mandarin name literally means "root from the Western seas." It is considered more yin than the Chinese ginseng and more gentle and cooling, with a particular affinity for the digestive system, lungs, and overall energy of the body. It manifests earth energy—sustaining, grounding, and strengthening for the body, emotions, and mind. Like the earth, ginseng's force enhances life and benefits the heart and spirit. Because it nourishes the yin and the fluids, American ginseng is commonly found in many formulas to treat deficient yin disharmony patterns: low-grade fevers, restlessness, irritability, weakness, and thirst. It nourishes the lung yin and so is used for coughing, slight fevers, thirst, and loss of voice. It also nourishes the nervous system and is administered in cases of fatigue, restlessness, insomnia, and exhaustion. American ginseng is found, like its Oriental cousin, in many tonic and strengthening formulas.

American ginseng roots, often 2 to 4 inches long, are slender and whitish. The authentic ginseng root has an unmistakable flavor. Different grades exist, as well as low-quality and even bogus roots. Many of the bottled products are inferior, few label the product adequately, and there is no way of knowing the size, age, or grade of the ginseng liquid, tablet, or powder. The trade of ginseng is poorly regulated. Dr. Albert Leung, an herbal researcher, advises that the buyer do what the Hong Kong wife does: "make a trip to the herbalist's, where you can buy the whole root." There you can compare different roots and begin to understand the different qualities, sizes, and ages. Liquid extracts of ginseng from China or America are sometimes quite good, and with these the quality of the ginseng can be judged to some degree by the taste.

There are many classic ginseng formulas, some commercially available. One ancient formula, developed originally by Taoist priests, is said to build the three vital treasures, Jing, Chi, and Shen, to create good health, a jovial personality, and an open heart. The longevity formula consists of equal parts of ginseng, he shou wu, lycium, schisandra, and asparagus root, simmered gently in water for an hour or two, and used two times daily for several weeks. Ginseng is a major herb of fu zhen therapy, which aims to improve overall health and prevent disease.

Modern efforts to standardize ginseng, to extract the most "active" elements, the ginsenosides, might have value in terms of research, but traditional herbalists feel that medicine made from the whole plant is best. Biochemist Albert Leung explains: "You have to take into account everything and how they work together, rather than just one aspect. . . . If you selectively extract the ginsenosides then you are leaving a lot of the root behind." This is not to say, however, that commercial ginseng extracts should not guarantee a minimum of ginsenosides, which are not found in some products.

Primary Uses. Increases energy, enhances the immune system, and strengthens the lungs; fatigue, weakness, dry cough, shallow breathing, no appetite, fatigue, adrenal exhaustion, insomnia, palpitations, and nervous exhaustion.

Doses. Extract, capsules, and powders, standard doses, twice daily. For medium-term use, several weeks, with a break. A common method is to chew pieces of the root or make a tea from the root pieces or powder. The tea or decoction can be taken 2 times a day for several days to several weeks, depending on the need and constitution of the person. American ginseng is milder than the Oriental and blends very well with astragalus.

Cautions. A safe, mild herb but one that should be used moderately during pregnancy and lactation with the guidance of an herbalist.

Complementary Remedies. Elecampane, astragalus, St. John's wort, and reishi.

CHINESE GINSENG
Panax schinseng

Ginseng, a small green herb, prefers the shady woods of cool green mountains, but nowadays Oriental wild ginseng is xceedingly rare. In the old days the aristocratic ginseng roots, from mature wild plants in secret stands, were considered more valuable than gold, and people would literally die for them. Secret ginseng cults flourished, and gangs of ginseng thieves were often thwarted with traps, poisons, and arrows. The aristocracy had their own tightly guarded ginseng reserves, and death was a common punishment for those thieves who tried to dig up the roots. The goal was to try to preserve patches of mature (more than seven years old) ginseng, a difficult goal because not only thieves threaten the ginseng but also fungus, moles, deer, and other pests.

In northern China, woodsmen once hunted the elusive ginseng. These rugged hunters, who lived a life of adventure and danger, would spend many lonely weeks in remote mountains, exposed to elements, wild animals, and fierce bandits who would kill them for their roots. During the time of the hunt, they would refrain from meat and sexual intercourse and prepare themselves with exercises and meditation. Sometimes they relied on their dreams for guidance about where to hunt.

However, today there are few places in the Orient where wild ginseng can be found. Ginseng is notoriously difficult to grow and takes a farmer of great skill and patience. For centuries ginseng has been cultivated under long, shaded canopies where it matures for seven or more years. Ginseng plantations are a major agricultural endeavor in Korea, where more than 70,000 people are employed to grow, maintain, and process this valuable plant. The roots, often preserved by steaming and soaking in date sugar and other herbs, are graded according to size. The larger, older roots are more valuable. The red ginseng has been cured; the straw-colored is natural. Inferior ginseng is quite common and can generally be spotted by the small, poor-quality roots. The ginseng expert knows the age, type, and source of the root by touch, taste, and smell.

There are still people in the modern world who claim ginseng is just an Oriental placebo, a statement that reflects deep cultural ignorance and bias. Ginseng has been prized by top-quality Oriental physicians for hundreds of years, and they have a track record that exceeds anyone in the West by hundreds of years. Because ginseng is an adaptogen, a holistic term not yet clearly understood by most Western doctors, it cannot be examined or tested like typical drugs. Nevertheless, research validating ginseng is compiling some substantial results, based on the study of ginsenosides (at least twelve have been identified at this time), one of the principal constituents of the plant. Constituents include a whole range of vitamins and minerals and the triterpene saponins, essential oils, and polysaccharides.

Therapeutic Benefits. In Oriental medicine this root is said to be sweet, warming, and restoring for vital energy and all systems—what herbalists now call an adaptogen. For the human body we see seven basic benefits of ginseng:

1. Benefits the stomach and digestive system.
2. Relaxes the nervous system and improves circulation.
3. Studies suggest that ginseng builds energy by supporting the pituitary and adrenal glands and metabolism.
4. There are indications that ginseng is a nonspecific mild stimulant to the immune system.
5. Three themes of current ginseng research: cancer prevention, lowering cholesterol, and alleviating menopausal symptoms.
6. All the effects indicate that ginseng is good for overworked, overstressed modern people suffering from lack of energy.
7. Ginseng is also said to promote wisdom!

First Aid. The extract or tea is used to revive the stressed out or weak.

Primary Uses. Fatigue, increase of stamina, recovery from illness and accident; problems of old age like memory loss. Ginseng enhances healing and improves resistance and concentration. Herbalists also recommend it for weak lungs with shortness of breath, weak digestion, agitated heart and spirit.

Health Promotion. Ginseng is one of the classic herbs to promote health but is most often found in formulas with synergistic herbs.

Doses. Extracts, capsules, and crude root, recommended doses. The German Commission E recommends a daily dose of 1 to 2 grams of Asian ginseng, divided into three portions. Standardized extracts of ginseng, which are more concentrated, should be taken according to recommendations, often 150 milligrams per day, specified with at least 2 percent ginsenosides. It is recommended that ginseng, like other adaptogens, not be taken continuously for months. One possibility is to use the remedy for 2 or 3 weeks, a break, and then possibly again.

A Chinese herbalist told me that the best form of ginseng is the fresh root. As that is hard for many people to acquire, the dried whole root is second best. This can be chewed. Slice off tiny pieces or slightly steam small sections, then eat. Roots can also be decocted at home, and the tea drunk several times daily. Ginseng is contained in countless Oriental formulas, some of which can be purchased as extracts, pills, or tablets. One of the most popular ginseng formulas, the "four gentleman concoction," contains ginseng, atractylodis, poria cocos (*fu ling*), and licorice, up to 9 grams of the first 3, and 6 of the licorice—available in prepared form.

Ginseng extracts, with a distinctive flavor, can be quite good, but many of the commercial ginseng tonics contain little ginseng. In other words, ginseng extracts should be purchased from a reputable company that specializes in herbal medicine. The Korean ginseng is said to be a little more "yang," or stimulating, than the Chinese, but both are most commonly used for people over forty.

Cautions. Ginseng is a safe healing plant but should be avoided by those with high blood pressure, fevers, or overactive nervous systems. Strong, active younger people should probably avoid this herb. Overused, or more accurately abused, ginseng can occasionally cause nervousness, irritability, insomnia, and agitation. Pregnant or lactating women should avoid this herb, unless specifically directed by an Oriental herbalist.

SIBERIAN GINSENG
Eleutherococcus senticosus
Ci wu ji

Siberian ginseng is not a true ginseng but a member of the large ginseng family, the Araliaceae. Nevertheless, this plant, found in Russia and China, is a useful adaptogen. Siberian ginseng, also called eleuthero, is an energy tonic intently studied and valued in Russia. Dr. Israel Brekhman, a Russian scientist, pioneered studies of Siberian ginseng; in 1961, he and his colleagues published a paper on this plant. At first they called it a stimulant and tonic, but on further reflection they coined the current term, *adaptogen*. An adaptogen is a substance that is relatively harmless and causes minimal disturbance in the physiological functions of the body; at the same time it must have a nonspecific action to modulate stress and improve performance under a wide variety of stressful conditions.

Studies in Russia and other countries have confirmed that Siberian ginseng is indeed an adaptogen. It maintains levels of energy and alertness under a wide variety of stressful conditions, including intense work, motion, heat, noise, and exercise. It increases mental alertness, overall energy, and quality of work under a variety of stressful conditions and athletic performance. It comes as no surprise that this herb has become a favorite of athletes, who use it and other herbs to improve their energy, endurance, and alertness. In Russia Siberian ginseng has been used by ordinary folk, factory workers, politicians, cosmonauts, ballet dancers, mine and mountain rescue workers, and Olympic athletes, as well as those recovering from shock, trauma, and surgery.

Recent studies are revealing some interesting facts about this unusual plant remedy, focusing on the examination of the eleutherosides and polysaccharides. Siberian ginseng assists patients recovering from chemotherapy and radiation. It also improves resistance and endurance and might even have some use in diverse conditions like Alzheimer's disease and the common cold.

First Aid. Recovery from trauma and accident.

Primary Uses. For conditions of tiredness from overwork and overstress. In addition, for people recovering from chronic disease, radiation, chemotherapy, and surgery—a use that it shares with other ginsengs. Siberian ginseng is helpful for the kind of arthritis that is sensitive to damp weather. Herbalists also use this herb for chronic fatigue and muscle pain.

Health Promotion. Like all adaptogens, Siberian ginseng is a health-promoting plant medicine and is best used conservatively for optimum results.

Doses. In liquid extract, 10 to 30 drops twice a day, depending on constitution and age. It can also be found in capsules, tablets, and synergistic formulas; can be taken for up to 4 to 6 weeks with a break before resuming.

Cautions. Pregnant women can use this herb, but those with very high blood pressure should avoid it.

GOLDENSEAL
Hydrastis canadensis

CHEROKEE MEDICINE

Goldenseal, one of the great Native American healing plants, is a therapeutic giant. Like ginseng, goldenseal is a small green herb that favors shady eastern forests; in the past decades it has been overpicked, making it an endangered plant. The medicine is prepared from the root and rhizome. Goldenseal was a popular medicine with many eastern tribes and was also commonly used as a dye and to paint faces, hence the common name *Indian dye*. It has a distinct yellow color and its root's surface is ridged with scarlike patterns, thus the name *goldenseal*. Cherokee Indians have traditionally valued goldenseal, using it for a variety of ailments, even cancer. Indians introduced this herb to Captain Meriwether Lewis of the famous Lewis and Clark expedition, who used it for sore inflamed eyes and mouth sores.

Health Benefits. Goldenseal, adopted by early pioneers and hunters, was applied to cuts, wounds, and insect bites. In 1852 Dr. John King, the great Eclectic physician, introduced this plant into a massive compendium of natural remedies, and from that time goldenseal was favored by the Eclectic physicians. In the nineteenth century, this herb was extremely popular in America, finding its way into the notorious patent medicines that flourished at the time—for example, Dr. Pierce's Golden Medical Discovery. While many claims for these popular medicines were exaggerated, if not absurd, some had therapeutic properties because they contained potent Indian medicines like goldenseal.

Traditionally goldenseal was used to detoxify the body,

and thus prevent and cure diseases of the lungs and digestive tract, and to prevent bleeding. Today, it is a major botanical medicine, primarily employed as a cleansing tonic in a variety of health conditions, particularly skin, stomach, respiratory, and lymphatic problems. A bitter-tasting medicine, goldenseal is considered cooling and astringent. It clears toxins, inflammations, and unwanted mucus secretions. Goldenseal's essential ingredient, berberine, displays broad spectrum antibiotic activity.

First Aid. Goldenseal powder is used for cuts, abrasions, and fungal infections.

Primary Uses. For everyday use: for sinusitis, colds, coughs, flu, and, in tiny doses, to promote healthy digestion. Herbalists prescribe goldenseal for these conditions as well as for bacterial and fungal infections, ulcers, skin problems, gastritis, canker sores, parasites, itching or burning skin, and coughs with thick yellow mucus. Goldenseal is also said to stimulate the liver and gallbladder and has potential in cysts, painful breasts, and sore lumps. It can be applied externally and in douches.

Health Promotion. This versatile herb is a major healer, but see the restrictions that follow. Goldenseal, in small doses—5 to 10 drops in water twice daily—for a few days, is a tonic for the digestive system.

Doses. Capsules, tablets, and extracts—recommended doses. Liquid extracts in small amounts, 5 to 15 drops in water or juice, 2 to 3 times a day, or in synergistic formulas as directed. Use minute quantities for small, thin, or delicate people. Children can take a few drops in water or juice several times a day, or 3x or 6x homeopathic pellets. The powder can be used for skin problems, the mouthwash for the gums and mouth. Goldenseal was once a main ingredient in skin ointments for wounds, growths, and ulcers. For a douche, dissolve 1 tablespoon of powder in a cup of warm water and allow to cool. Goldenseal is an herb to take for the short term, and not for medical problems without medical advice.

Cautions. Contraindicated in pregnancy, in nursing, and for those with high blood pressure. Goldenseal is a safe natural medicine when used judiciously.

Complementary Remedies. Barberry, echinacea; osha and lomatium for viral diseases.

Note. An informative article on goldenseal: Steven Foster, "Goldenseal, *Hydrastis canadensis*," Botanical Series no. 309 (Austin, TX: American Botanical Council, 1991).

GOTU KOLA
Centella asiatica

AYURVEDIC HEALER

Gotu kola, also known as Indian pennywort, is one of the premier medicines of Ayurveda, the indigenous medicine of the huge Indian subcontinent. There it has been valued for hundreds of years, as well as in tropical Africa, Sri Lanka, Indonesia, and China. Gotu kola is a common plant in the tropics, described as a low creeping weed that lusts after water. Legend has it that elephants also lust after gotu kola— the reason why, according to folk healers, they live a long, intelligent life. In Asia there is a common saying about gotu kola: "Eat two leaves a day and keep old age away." In India gotu kola has been known as a longevity herb that is particularly restorative for the nervous system. It is also well

known in Oriental medicine, and in the modern era it is recognized by global herbalism. Traditionally, gotu kola is also
used for skin diseases like leprosy and psoriasis. This herb
should not be confused with kola nut, a plant that contains
caffeine.

Health Benefits. Gotu kola is, nevertheless, a controversial
herbal medicine, because it is a relatively new medicine in the
West and has two different uses in Asiatic medical systems.
On the one hand, it is universally claimed as a healer of the
skin, an application supported by modern research. For this
purpose it is prescribed for wounds, varicose veins, ulcers, and
skin inflammations. On the other hand, it has a venerable reputation as a versatile adaptogen. In central Asia it has been
touted as a nerve and brain tonic, used for memory loss, senility, premature aging, and to promote longevity. In fact, one
of the names for this herb in India is *Brahma*, the name of
the supreme reality, and it is said to be a favorite tea of med-
itating yogis. Many Ayurvedic physicians call gotu kola the
premier restorative herb of Ayurveda, a substantial claim
when you consider that they are intimately familiar with
hundreds of medicinal plants.

Ayurvedic medicine, like the Chinese, most often prescribes adaptogenic herbs like gotu kola with other herbs, in
formulas that have been valued for centuries. Therefore,
more research is needed to determine the single and
polypharmic effects of gotu kola. Modern research has yet to
catch up on this herb, but to some degree it has been examined, and there are some interesting developments in this
sleuth work—chasing after the legend of one of Asia's premier tonic plants.

The dreaded leprosy, an insidious degenerative disease, is

not impervious to the action of gota kola—not that gotu kola will supplant modern drugs that work very well for this bacterial-induced disease. A study published in the English journal *Nature* explained that the bacterium that causes leprosy has a waxy coating to protect it from the immune system. A chemical in gotu kola dissolves this coating, exposing the bacterium to the attack of immune cells. Studies indicate, too, that gotu kola promotes circulation to the legs, that gotu kola cream can relieve itching red skin problems, and that it accelerates the healing of wounds, ulcers, and cuts. Gotu kola, it appears, also has mild sedative properties, thus its use for calming the nerves, inducing relaxation, and even promoting better health.

First Aid. Gotu kola cream or poultices are used for cuts, itchy red rashes, minor burns, and to promote the healing of scars.

Primary Uses. Herbalists use this herb to improve the memory, to clean the blood, to calm the nerves, and as an adaptogen. Gotu kola increases energy and is valued for the aging, depression, nervousness, fatigue, and learning problems, as well as ulcers, psoriasis, varicose veins, and other skin problems. It also is said to tone the heart and lift the spirits.

Health Promotion. Gotu kola quite clearly has the potential to promote better health.

Doses. A tea; follow recommended doses for extracts and capsules. Gotu kola is now commonly found in excellent formulas, particularly with ginkgo. Some herbalists recommend standardized extracts of gotu kola to ensure active constituents. Do not use this herb for the long term without professional advice.

Cautions. Contraindicated during pregnancy and nursing. Topical applications have been known to create itching—discontinue use.

GREEN TEA
Camellia sinensis

HEALING BEVERAGE

After water, tea is the most common beverage in the world. Coffee comes third. Most people do not consider coffee or tea herbal medicines, but they are potent medicinal plants. Each day millions of cups of these beverages are consumed. They have had a profound effect on the life of humankind, not only because of their gentle stimulus and good taste, but because much energy has gone into growing, preparing, and using these two herbs. It is not an exaggeration to say that wars have been started on account of tea and coffee. Certainly, they have had an immense influence on the history of many countries. England, for example, developed a lasting taste for tea in the seventeenth century, and today the average English person cannot do without four o'clock teatime. And as we all know, tea has had its influence on American history: when the English tried to raise the tax on tea in the American colonies, they prompted the famous Boston Tea Party.

Because the tea had to be imported from China at great cost, the English began their own plantations in India, Sri Lanka, and other tropical nations, an endeavor that altered the history of several nations. So successful were these plantations that China soon lost its dominance in the tea trade.

Today, tea is the major cash crop on the island of Sri Lanka. Major tea plantations also exist in China, Japan, Kenya, India, and Indonesia, providing enough tea (2.5 million tons a year) to satisfy the needs of the world's population.

Both China and India vie for credit for the origin of tea. The Chinese claim that the legendary leader Shen Nong introduced agriculture and medicine into ancient China about 3000 B.C. One of the herbal medicines he brought to humankind was green tea. The Indians claim that the Buddha brought tea to China, even though no evidence exists that he went there. Apparently the Buddha was outraged when on his pilgrimage through China he fell asleep inappropriately, breaking a vow. In rage he tore off his eyelids and threw them to the ground! The eyelids sprouted as tea plants that had the potential to banish fatigue.

Tea, a small evergreen tree that is cultivated as a shrub, generally thrives in tropical mountains where the temperature is mild and the moisture plentiful. The tidy, green, lush rows are beautiful to observe in countries like Japan where tea is cultivated like a Zen garden. Tea leaves are best harvested by hand because machinery tends to bruise or rip the delicate leaves. Sri Lanka, a lovely island with moist green hills, produces an abundant crop of world-class tea. There one can see lines of colorfully dressed women patiently picking the leaves, wearing straw hats to protect themselves from the sun and large woven collecting baskets around their waists.

Around the planet, different kinds of tea are cultivated like fine wines, and some blends are now world famous for their distinctive flavors: Oolong, English breakfast, Earl Grey, and many others. Often a special process flavors these famous blends. Earl Grey, for example, is blended with the oil of bergamot, a citrus tree that grows in India and Italy.

Health Benefits. Tea contains less caffeine than coffee and is generally considered more healthful, especially green tea, which has been popular in Asia for thousands of years. Green tea is milder than the more common black teas, but both come from the same leaves. A light steaming (or roasting) produces green tea. It is prepared from the fresh-cut green leaf, a process that prevents oxidation and prevents key compounds in the leaf from decomposing. The health benefits of green teas are now verified by scientific research. Green tea is rich in compounds called polyphenols, powerful antioxidants that have some surprising health benefits. The green tea polyphenols, contained to a lesser degree in black tea, are potent antioxidants that protect against degeneration and disease, most notably cancer. A number of studies have indicated that green tea can indeed protect against cancer by inhibiting the formation of carcinogens. Green tea contains antibacterial properties, improves the cholesterol profile, and protects the blood vessels from atherosclerosis. Green tea contains caffeine (a modest amount), lignans, amino acids, vitamins, organic acids, protein, and chlorophyll.

Primary Uses. A healthy and relaxing beverage, also used as an adjunct in cancer therapy, to prevent tooth decay, and to promote health of the blood vessels.

Health Promotion. General use to promote good health.

Doses. This safe herb is ingested as tea, up to 3 cups a day. The Japanese drink green tea with their meals, said to be a particularly advantageous way of ingesting it. Green tea is found as a food supplement in capsules, extracts, and synergistic formulas.

Cautions. Those sensitive to caffeine. Pregnant and nursing mothers should consult their physician before taking medicinal potions of any caffeinated beverage.

GREENS: BROCCOLI, KALE, AND OTHERS, PRIMARILY THE CRUCIFEROUS GREEN LEAFY VEGETABLES

GREEN PHARMACY

It might surprise some people to see green vegetables like broccoli, kale, and cabbage called power herbs, because in our culture green vegetables are not generally considered medicinal. However, it would be no exaggeration to call them the ultimate in green pharmacy. Recent scientific studies are validating the traditional claims of these especially nourishing foods. In fact, I recently read a study that indicated that folic acid (particularly rich in greens) can slow the progress of senility and Alzheimer's disease. In herbal medicine greens are considered nourishing for the whole body, especially the blood, the immune, and the digestive systems. They contain valuable vitamins and minerals as well as antioxidants—even anticancer properties. Without doubt, from the mouth to stomach to the intestines the greens protect against serious degenerative diseases.

In traditional systems of medicine—whether of China, India, or Europe—food has always been the first line of defense against disease. Until very recently contemporary medicine put food medicine on the back, back shelf. The prevalent dogma was that food had little role in the prevention of disease. During the brave new era of synthetic drug

supremacy—from the beginning of the 1900s to the 1990s—
physicians who put food first were often ignored, laughed at,
or even worse put on trial. A case in point was the brilliant
German physician Dr. Max Gerson, who moved to America
to escape the Nazis in the 1930s. Dr. Gerson developed a
comprehensive nutritional program for cancer (and other
diseases), but he was hounded by his colleagues and their
professional organizations, despite his impeccable character.
Dr. Albert Schweitzer called him "one of the most eminent
geniuses in medical history." The American Cancer Society
roundly criticized Dr. Gerson and did not recognize the
nutritional link of cancer prevention until the 1980s. Only
today can we begin to appreciate the genius and courage of
this medical pioneer, as research validates nutritional facts at
an amazing rate. We are in a renaissance of nutritional
research, and it is becoming readily apparent that nutrition
does have a major role to play in preventative medicine. Even
more difficult to accept is that nutrition has a major role to
play in the actual treatment of major diseases: arthritis, cancer, high blood pressure, and many others. For example,
recently a study revealed that a diet high in vegetables, fruits,
and fiber was as effective as prescription drugs in controlling
many cases of high blood pressure. This radical information
would have been laughed at a mere decade ago.

We all need the carbohydrates, proteins, essential fatty
acids, fiber, vitamins, enzymes, and minerals contained in
grains, meats, fruit, and vegetables. But for the purposes of this
book I can say one group of foods can be elevated to the status of power herbs: these are the leafy green vegetables. In his
food therapy Dr. Gerson often included fresh juices or broths
made from green vegetables. These would be consumed each

day by his cancer patients. Research has validated the cancer-inhibitory power of leafy greens, particularly the cruciferous twelve. These twelve vegetables all have flowers with four petals that to botanic observers resembled a cross—hence cruciferous. They all share common phytochemicals that inhibit tumor formation and counteract some of the destruction caused by carcinogens. They also play a major role in the treatment of other diseases like arthritis, heart disease, and hypertension.

The cruciferous twelve are: *broccoli, Brussels sprouts, cabbage, cauliflower, watercress, horseradish, kale, kohlrabi, mustard, radish, rutabaga,* and *turnip greens*.

In traditional systems of food culture, such as the Italian and Oriental, greens (and of course other vegetables) play a major role. Interestingly enough, most traditional forms of diet are loaded with healthy foods that inhibit high cholesterol, cancer, heart disease, and arthritis—major problems of modern Western people. To take one example, the traditional Italian cuisine consists of garlic, olive oil, greens, pasta, basil, oregano, tomatoes, and fish—all recognized for a variety of healthful properties. Tomatoes contain a powerful antioxidant, lycopene, that is now believed to be a cancer preventative. Garlic is a superfood and one of the power herbs of this book. Olive oil, one of the healthiest kitchen oils, is loaded with nutritional benefits. Basil, oregano, and other common Italian herbs are valuable medicines in their own right. The traditional Italian diet, like that of many other countries, was founded, without any academic experts, on a solid nutritional basis.

Greens are a rich storehouse of good health and nutrition. Take one humble vegetable as an example: *kale*. In America the green leafy kale is often only served as a decoration to meat and fish dishes and then finds its way into the garbage. A pity, because kale, like all the cruciferous vegetables, is a storehouse of healthy nutrition and disease-preventing antioxidants. It is an excellent source of vegetable fiber good for the intestines and whole body and a bountiful source of one of the most antioxidants, the carotenoids. Kale has twice the amount of carotenoids found in spinach. It has more beta-carotene, a precursor of vitamin A, than an equivalent weight of carrots. If that were not enough, kale is a rich source of chlorophyll, the green pigment, which is also a healthful substance. Collard greens, a favorite green of Southern blacks, is a similar superfood. These greens appear to reduce the risk of cancer by promoting enzymes that help to detoxify carcinogens. Sulforaphane, a health-promoting antioxidant, is one of the potent constituents of these greens. In her book *Powerfoods*, Dr. Stephanie Beling calls leafy greens the preeminent cancer-protecting foods, rich in indoles and sulforaphanes that block cancer-causing agents from reaching the healthy cells.[17]

People who consume large amounts of vegetables like kale, cabbage, and mustard greens have lower rates of gastrointestinal, esophageal, stomach, lung, colon, oral, and throat cancers—perhaps all cancers. Cruciferous vegetables are especially linked to lower rates of bowel, prostrate, and bladder cancer.[18] Those who eat leafy greens, even if they are smokers, can expect a lower rate of lung cancer. Need we say more about these superfoods, the greens? Yes. The humble

17. Stephanie Beling, *Powerfoods* (New York: HarperCollins, 1997), p. 68.

18. Jean Carper, *The Food Pharmacy* (Toronto/New York: Bantam, 1988), p. 221.

cabbage is a longevity food of some distinction. Cabbage has numerous phytochemicals that inhibit cancer, as well as antibiotic and antiviral properties. People who eat cabbage regularly have lower rates of colon cancer, even of all diseases![19] Cabbage, however, might be harmful when eaten in excess as a salty pickled food.

Health Promotion. These greens are quite obviously foods we should eat every day. They help to prevent arthritis, cancer, and innumerable bowel problems and are basically good for every major organ and function of the body, particularly the lungs, liver, blood, and intestines.

Doses. It is sensible to eat greens and other vegetables every day, preferably 2 times a day. *Cooked or raw?* While it is true that cooking destroys some nutrients, it also makes others more available for assimilation. Raw might be preferable in the final analysis, but some people cannot efficiently digest raw foods. Eat your greens cooked and raw. Without doubt greens are better when prepared fresh and when possible grown organically. Recent research has demonstrated that broccoli and other greens are quite variable in quality, depending on where they are grown, when they are harvested, and how they are transported and stored. Sulforaphane and other critical constituents can vary. The classic herbalists have always been very careful about the growing and harvesting of herbs, a tendency that is beginning to be validated by current research in sulforaphane levels in different batches of broccoli.

For certain diseases and people, special extracts or juices of greens are highly beneficial. Cancer patients, for example,

19. Ibid., p. 151.

might drink raw juices of greens mixed with carrot juice each day. Cabbage juice can heal ulcers. For people recovering from any long-term degenerative disease, green food supplementation is not only a good idea, it is an excellent one.

Complementary Vegetables. Carrots, beets, onions, and radishes (all kinds) also protect against cancer and other degenerative diseases.

Note. For more guidance about healthy diet, see *Natural Health, Natural Medicine,* by Andrew Weil.

HAWTHORN
Crataegus spp.

HEART REMEDY

Hawthorn is a small spiny tree or shrub native to Europe, where the blossoms and fruit have been valued as a medicine for many centuries. The common name *hawthorn* is a corruption of *hedgethorn;* it was used in Germany to divide plots of land. Lovely delicate white blossoms adorn the tree in springtime, and when ripe the fruit is a brilliant red. The medicine is prepared from the flowers, fruit, and leaves and is one of the major herbal remedies for the heart and cardiovascular system.

This durable tree is rich in folklore, a veritable treasure of tales, poems, and legends. One legend states that the thorns of the tree were used to crown the head of Jesus. Traditionally hawthorn was one of the major sacred trees of Europe. Its overall popularity can be seen in the many strange names that have been used over the centuries: *mayflower, mayblossom, whitethorn, quick, haw, hazels, gazels, halves hagthorn, ladies meat*, and *bread and cheese tree*. The famous Pilgrim ship the *Mayflower* was named after this tree. Formerly the hard wood, renowned for its fine grain, was made into small items like music boxes.

Species of hawthorn can be found in Asia and the Middle East. The Chinese use their species of hawthorn for digestive problems, particularly for sluggish digestion and abdominal distension, but they also value the remedy for unblocking the arteries and to treat heart pain. American Indians also use hawthorn. Interestingly enough, the herbal physicians of nineteen-century America, the Eclectics, were well aware of the healing properties of this plant. As late as 1922 Dr. Felter said: "There can be no question as to its value as a tonic to the heart muscle."[20] Sadly, however, hawthorn and other herbal medicines have been neglected by conventional medicine. Heart disease, which can be prevented to some degree by these herbs, is the number-one killer in America.

Health Benefits. Today hawthorn is a power herb of some repute and much clinical usage. Its medicinal properties, heavily researched, primarily stem from compounds called procyanidins and flavonoids. In Europe it is recognized as a safe and gentle heart tonic and is used to treat irregular heartbeat, angina pectoris, heart palpitations, arteriosclerosis, and valvular heart disease. It improves circulation of the blood and the health of the blood vessels and heart. Very valuable in problems of the elderly, hawthorn is considered by herbalists to be an excellent preventative medicine. It also has some

20. Harvey Wickes Felter, *The Eclectic Materia Medica* (Portland, OR: Eclectic Medical Publications, 1985), p. 326.

use for sleeplessness, especially for insomnia that develops from too much thinking and nervousness.

The most famous modern drug for the heart is digitalis, originally made from the lovely foxglove plant; while an effective remedy, this prescription drug must be administered with skill and caution. Other herbs for the heart include lily of the valley and hawthorn. In Oriental medicine, the heart organ is said to be more than an extraordinary muscle. It is called the king, or queen if you're a woman, of the body, radiating warmth, feeling, and beneficence. It is an interesting fact that most of the valuable natural remedies for the heart are made from distinctive flowering plants.

Primary Uses. Herbalists use hawthorn alone and with other herbs for insomnia, nervousness, difficult breathing, blood pressure irregularities, hypertension, palpitations, organic degenerative heart diseases, angina, arteriosclerosis, irregularities of heartbeat, and hypertension.

Health Promotion. A major preventative remedy; one of the great remedies for elderly people along with ginkgo, garlic, olive oil, and ginseng.

Doses. Extracts, capsules, tablets, and synergistic formulas. As with many herbal medicines, infusions or tinctures made from the fresh flowers, berries, and leaves are the best preparation of this remedy. Hawthorn is a safe remedy that should be taken for some time to achieve its full benefit. In Germany, flower and leaf preparations are recommended, 160 milligrams per day, divided into 2 portions.

Cautions. It is strongly recommended that heart problems not be self-diagnosed or treated without the advice of a physician.

HE SHOU WU
Polygonum multiflorum

ORIENTAL LONGEVITY TONIC

He shou wu, commercially called fo ti in America, is a famous longevity tonic in the Orient. There is a proverbial story related to its discovery in China. During the Tang dynasty, there was a man called He Shou Wu who became very depressed one day because he hadn't been able to conceive any children. He was fifty-eight and had been impotent for many years. On this day he drank himself into a stupor and stumbled up a hillside where he promptly feel into a deep sleep. When he awoke the next morning, he saw a vine growing next to him that sparked his curiosity. Like most Chinese at the time he was knowledgeable about medicinal herbs, but he did not know this one. He dug up the root, took it home, and showed it to an old herbalist near his village. The herbalist said that this particular root was a very powerful tonic that could restore strength and health. Prematurely aged, He Shou Wu decided to consume a tea made from this medicine every day for three months. Soon he started to feel stronger and regained his virility, and in time his gray hair darkened. He raised several children and grew to be 130 years old. In this story, the effects of this medicine are exaggerated, but he shou wu remains one of the premier tonics of Oriental medicine.

He shou wu, a twining vine that grows up to 6 feet long, produces a bounty of tiny flowers (*multiflorum*). In China, like most bindweeds, it grows like a weed almost anywhere, but in America it is a rare ornamental plant. The medicine, made from the root, is harvested in the fall. The large roots are then cleaned, cut into pieces, and dried. It is known as *kashuu* in Japan, where it is also renowned. The processed root is a little sweet, astringent, and slightly warm. In Chinese medicine it is said to strengthen the liver and kidneys and nourish the vital essence (*jing*) and the blood. It is used primarily for deficient yin, a pattern of symptoms including prematurely graying hair, weak lower back and knees, soreness in the extremities, insomnia, dizziness, impotence, and restlessness. It nourishes people who are passing their half-century mark, particularly those who have burnt the candle at both ends—in other words, the modern Western man or woman. He shou wu is reputed to improve the sex life of both sexes, administered by itself or in formulas for impotence and infertility. Whether he shou wu can truly turn gray hair black, I cannot vouch for, but there is no doubt that the venerable tradition of Oriental medicine respects this plant medicine. He shou wu is a valuable tonic for Western people. Research indicates that it lowers blood pressure and cholesterol levels. Possibly this root can inhibit tumor formation—more research is necessary.

Primary Uses. Oriental herbalists use this herb for fatigue, depression, sexual weakness, lack of stamina, signs of premature aging, premature graying, high blood pressure, and high cholesterol.

Health Promotion. He shou wu is a major longevity tonic in Oriental medicine. While it can be used by itself, it is often found in synergistic formulas with other power herbs like ginseng and dong quai. A safe natural medicine that should be taken for some time; as with most health-promoting herbs, it is better to pause a few weeks, or consult an Oriental herbalist.

Doses. Liquid extract, capsules, and tablets can now be

purchased in America. Standard doses are for several weeks or more, or as directed by a health professional. For decocting at home, the darker the root the better, and the neatly sliced roots are usually superior. This herb is often blended with ginseng, dong quai, ligustrum, and others. Shou Wu Chih, a he shou wu formula, is a commercial extract available in herbal shops.

KAVA KAVA
Piper methysticum

POLYNESIAN EXOTIC

As we go around our globe we discover major herbs from every region, a few of which have been elevated to international status. Kava, a therapeutic plant from the Pacific islands, is not included in this book for geographic or curiosity reasons. This major herbal medicine has been thoroughly examined by modern science. It is a valuable remedy for modern people because it reduces nervous excitement and stress without impeding mental clarity, a rarity in medicine. Clinically this herb is used by itself or in synergistic formulas for stress, anxiety, and sleeplessness.

Oceania is a vast and diverse area of island communities, including Micronesia, Melanesia, and Polynesia. Prior to the arrival of Europeans in the nineteenth century, this region was one of the few of this planet where people did not use alcoholic beverages. They did, however, possess a magical plant, kava, one they greatly cherished. Often used on special and religious occasions, this herb produces calmness and promotes sociability. Traditionally these island people are some of the happiest and friendliest in the world. The first European to describe kava was the pioneering British sailor Captain James Cook, who traversed the Pacific region several times. Each island has its legend related to the discovery of this divine plant.

In his essays on Polynesia, Robert W. Williamson relates the following Samoan story. One day Tangaloa came down from heaven with two assistants. To feed their master, the assistants went fishing with their hands, in the days before nets and hooks. The assistants caught a fish and brought it to the god, who wanted to enjoy his repast with the divine nectar, kava. As there was no kava on earth, he sent his help back to heaven to bring back a root, but by mistake they brought back a whole plant. Tangaloa scattered the extra parts of the plant over the earth, and there they took root. To make the kava liquid he needed water—it rained—and to prepare the nectar the assistants brought a bowl, a strainer, and a cup. This is how the gods introduced the kava ceremony to the island people.

An attractive shrub, this hardy perennial produces a root that is knotty and thick, and rich in what biochemists believe is the most active ingredient, kava lactones. However, the crude extract of the root is believed to produce the most effective sedative. In other words, like many natural remedies, this one is best when used whole. Kava kava has an interesting history in the Polynesian cultures, most often considered a sacred plant and utilized in ceremonies and social functions. Even visiting celebrities and politicians have been served the traditional kava brew: Pope Paul, Hillary Clinton, Lady Bird Johnson, and many others. The eminent pharmacologist Louis Lewin noted in 1886: "When the mixture [of kava] is not too strong, the subject attains a happy unconcern, well-being and contentment, free from physical or psychological excitement."[21]

Kava is not addictive or toxic like excess alcohol; it does not lead to depression or anger. In fact, sleep is often the worst result of overindulging in kava. Furthermore, kava does not alter the senses or psyche like marijuana or peyote. One does not lose contact with one's self; on the contrary, one becomes quite content with one's enhanced sense of well-being. Kava ceremonies do not result in disorderly conduct or hangovers. This plant acts unlike any natural or synthetic substance known to humanity, and it does not depress mental functions or seriously impact driving or operating heavy equipment— unless, of course, it is abused, or mixed with alcohol. It is quite possible that kava influences the ancient part of the brain, the limbic system, the primary seat of the emotions.

Primary Uses. Restlessness, insomnia, nervous anxiety, and muscle tension. The herb, also a mild diuretic, is now recognized by the German Commission E as a safe, effective medicine.

Doses. Extract: 10 to 30 drops in water, most often used before going to bed; also capsules and tablets. For insomnia it works well in synergistic formulas, often with valerian, another power herb.

Cautions. While kava is a safe herbal remedy, it should only be used short-term when it is needed. If a person exceeds recommended doses it could impair judgment—a special caution

21. Louis Lewin, *Phantastica: Narcotic and Stimulating Drugs, Their Use and Abuse* (London: Routledge and Kegan Paul, 1964).

for drivers—and it should not be mixed with excess alcohol, chemical sedatives, or psychoactive drugs. Possible effects from long-term use include skin symptoms and dryness. Pregnant and lactating women should avoid kava, as should people diagnosed with endogenous depression.

LICORICE
Glycyrrhiza glabra

THERAPEUTIC CANDY

Everyone has heard of licorice, but few know that it is a major Oriental herb found in countless herbal formulas. Known primarily as a flavorizer and candy in the West, licorice is a versatile healer. Licorice complements and enhances the action of other more famous herbs, accounting for its immense popularity in Oriental herbalism. However, licorice can stand well on its own as a power herb, hence its inclusion in this book. The major source of licorice in China is a species called G. *uralensis*. In the sixteenth century, licorice was mentioned in the famous Chinese herbal *Shen Nong Ben Cao Jing* in the superior class of herbs. The European licorice (G. *glabra*) is an acceptable substitute. Constituents of licorice include coumarins, flavonoids (at least twenty-five), terpenoids, volatile oils (at least eighty), amino acids, lignans, starches, sugars, and sterols. Glycyrrhizin, the most well-known constituent, is partly responsible for licorice's anti-inflammatory effects.

Health Benefits. In Oriental medicine licorice is said to invigorate the digestive organs, enhance the vital energy, alleviate coughs, and clear away heat and phlegm. It reduces pain, convulsions, and spasms and is also a powerful detoxifier—thus its importance in today's world. Highly regarded in the Orient, licorice is said to enhance energy and beauty. In India, China, and many other countries, licorice has an ancient use as a cough medicine.

Primary Uses. Herbalists use licorice alone and in formulas for coughs, sore throats, fatigue, asthma, swelling with pain, sores, and hepatitis and to alleviate symptoms of food poisoning. Chinese studies indicate that licorice is an excellent remedy for stomach or intestinal ulcers. It is an adrenal stimulant—the source of its venerable tonic qualities—and another important herb for people detoxifying from alcohol and drugs.

Health Promotion. By itself licorice is not an herb to take for a long time, but it is an important health-promoting herb in Chinese herbalism.

Doses. Decoction, capsules, and extracts, recommended doses, and can be taken in deglycyrrhizinated (DGL) doses to prevent water retention; otherwise the whole herb is preferred. A simple tonic can be prepared with ginseng and licorice: equal proportions, simmered gently for an hour and drunk daily for a few weeks.

Cautions. For those patients with high blood pressure or with problems of water retention. Instead, they can take the deglycrrhizinated licorice. Lactating and pregnant women should avoid licorice or seek medical advice.

LIGUSTRUM
Ligustrum lucidum
Nu-zhen-zi

ELIXIR OF YOUTH

An illustrious Oriental herbal medicine, ligustrum is beginning to make its way into America. A member of the famed
olive family, this common bushy plant is well known to gardeners because a related species grows in America and is
formed into hedges—the privet. The Chinese privet, notable
for its shiny evergreen leaves, can be found in the southern
United States. Worldwide there are about fifty species of
ligustrum, especially in Asia and Europe, but even as far-flung
as Australia.

In China, where it is a common shrub and small tree, ligustrum has been praised for many centuries. First mentioned in
the primary class of drugs in the *Shen Nong Ben Cao Jing* almost
two thousand years ago, it has appeared in most of the major
Oriental herbals since that time. Different parts of the plant
have been converted into medicine, but the major portion is
the small blue-black fruit, which is harvested in late fall and
allowed to dry, often mixed with a little honey, and steamed.
Traditionally, this remedy was well respected by Taoist priests
and martial artists, considered an elixir to promote long life,
health, and vigor, and often combined with other power herbs
like dong quai, he shou wu, and rehmannia.

Health Benefits. As a healing plant ligustrum is somewhat
similar to astragalus, also a power herb. They are both what
could loosely be called tonics—adaptogens that nourish the
whole body. In Oriental medicine ligustrum is a major yin
tonic, indicating that it nourishes the body on a deep level,

particularly in times of stress and transition. It is prescribed for a disharmony pattern known as yin deficiency of the liver and kidney, very common in busy modern people. This pattern produces symptoms like ringing in the ears, forgetfulness, dizziness, restlessness, premature gray hair, low back pain, poor sleep, and tiredness. Like astragalus, this herb is a gentle stimulant for the immune system, often prescribed to patients undergoing chemotherapy and radiation. Research has indicated several important properties: it is healthy for the blood vessels and heart and has antibacterial properties and may inhibit cancer. This nutritive herb also contains minerals, vitamins, and antioxidants.

Primary Uses. For nervous stress; immune stimulant; and adaptogen. See also the symptoms under *Health Benefits*.

Health Promotion. Most definitely an herb that is beneficial for modern people, comparable to other Oriental power herbs, he shou wu, ginseng, astragalus, and rehmannia.

Doses. The fruits can be decocted. Also extracts, pills, capsules, and synergistic formulas. This is considered a safe herb that can be taken for some time, often twice daily or as recommended by an herbalist. Ligustrum is one of the ingredients in the most common Oriental formula for women, "four substance soup," which also contains the power herbs dong quai and rehmannia (plus peony root—a major uterine tonic).

Cautions. Caution with diarrhea or chilly, weak patients. Otherwise a safe, nontoxic herb.

MILK THISTLE
Silybum marianum

HERBAL POWERHOUSE

Milk thistle, also known as St. Mary's thistle, is a potent healer much recommended for modern people. The use of this power herb, one of the stellar medicines of the European botanical tradition, has been substantiated by much scientific research. Milk thistle is one of many thistles and shares a place in herbal medicine with its relative, blessed or holy thistle, with which it should not be confused.

This tall handsome plant is considered by many to be a plain weed. It deserves more recognition for its beauty. Milk thistle bears the typical wavy spiny leaves of many thistles, but the glossy deep green leaves are decorated with curious white veins, and the tall stalk is topped by a lovely tuft of blue flowers. The plant has been valued in Europe since Roman times.

In 1694 the English herbalist Westmacott wrote this about milk thistle: "It is a friend to the liver and the blood: the prickles cut off, they were formally used to be boiled in spring and eaten with other herbs; but as the world decays, so doth the use of the good old things and others more delicate and less virtuous brought in."[22] Ah, poor Mr. Westmacott, he would be really disappointed if he were living today.

Health Benefits. A traditional name of this plant is *Our Lady's thistle*. An old tradition states that the milk-white veins originated from the milk of the Virgin Mary, who once fed on this plant. Nicholas Culpeper placed milk thistle under the dominion of Jupiter, which represents opening and

22. Grieve, *A Modern Herbal*, p. 797.

cleansing and naturally is associated with that Jupiterian organ, the liver. European herbalists see this plant as a powerful healer of the liver: softening, draining, cleansing, clearing obstructions (stones and fats), and ridding toxins. Interesting, too, is the traditional association of the plant with women, particularly the uterus, menstrual cramps, and delayed menses. Like many liver remedies, milk thistle also moves the bowels and prevents the formation of stones.

In the eighteen and nineteenth centuries, physicians respectful of botanical remedies used this thistle. Johann G. Rademacher, a German physician of the early nineteenth century, displayed a profound understanding of herbal medicines. He developed a preparation of milk thistle from the seeds, *Tinctura Cardui Mariae Rademacher,* an effective remedy still available in Europe. The American Eclectics also valued milk thistle, recognizing that it was a major liver remedy. In modern times milk thistle was forgotten outside the circles of botanical or homeopathic doctors. Recently, this neglect changed dramatically in Europe when scientists extracted an active principle, silymarin, from the seed and tested it extensively. The results were no less than astounding and more than validated centuries of use by herbalists. Silymarin protects and stimulates liver cells and is even used in Europe to heal the liver from mushroom poisoning and chemical toxins. The German Commission E recognizes milk thistle's unique role in medicine.

Because of its beneficial effect on the liver, milk thistle is especially valuable in our hectic modern era of rampant stress and chemical pollution. The liver, a very vital organ, detoxifies the blood of wastes and toxins. In the modern world the liver is a very busy organ indeed. Milk thistle is not only a useful healer for recovering alcoholics, drug addicts, and people who have had hepatitis, it can also be used by many of us as an occasional cleanser and tonic. Most often it is combined with other herbs, foods, and vitamins, particularly in a liver-cleansing program. Valued by many botanical doctors, milk thistle assists in the treatment of cancer patients, particularly those patients who participate in the rigorous program of chemotherapy or radiation.

Primary Uses. Heals the liver and gallbladder; headaches, nausea, mental depression, and dizziness—from torpid, overworked liver. Cirrhosis, hepatitis, the long-term effects of poisoning, gallstones, colic, skin rashes, stones, varicose veins, and sluggish bowel movement. Herbalists also have used this herb to stimulate milk production in nursing women and for menstrual problems.

Health Promotion. Undoubtedly milk thistle is a prime herb for health promotion, especially for those who have been exposed to drugs, chemicals, and excess alcohol.

Doses. Extract of milk thistle is excellent; also found in capsules, tablets, and synergistic formulas. Standardized doses are available, clearly labeled with the active constituent, silymarin, often up to 420 milligrams divided into 3 doses daily for up to 6 to 8 weeks, and then reduced to half the amount. By any standards, a safe herb.

Complementary Remedies. Schisandra, barberry, dandelion, goldenseal, osha, red clover, and burdock.

MYRRH
Commiphora molmol

ARABIC HEALING RESIN

One could mention few medicinal herbs with such a rich and varied history as myrrh. All around the planet, myrrh has been valued for thousands of years: by Egyptians, Romans, Chinese, Europeans, Africans, and Arabians. Arabia is the source of the tree from which the healing resin is collected. Myrrh grows on dry plateaus on the edge of the Arabian Peninsula as well as in Sudan and East Africa. Seasonally, Bedouins come to slash the tree bark, releasing a flow of white resin, which is then collected and dried. Remarkably, trade in this resin goes back to the days of the Bible. Myrrh was one of the gifts the wise men brought to the baby Jesus. Much lore and fable revolve around myrrh, but at the core of it all one finds a potent medicinal substance now verified by modern science.

The clear, fragrant gum resin of the myrrh tree has been used for thousands of years as a medicine, incense, ingredient in cosmetics and perfumes, fumigant, and for embalming. An Egyptian papyrus almost four thousand years old mentions the use of this therapeutic resin. The Egyptians rightfully valued the aroma of burning myrrh. On the walls of a temple a story is told that Amon, a god, told Queen Hatsheput in an oracle to plant myrrh trees around his temple. The queen ordered an expedition to the legendary land of Punt where the myrrh tree could be found. Ships ventured south to the territory of Punt, possibly modern Somaliland, where they encountered a strange tribe of black people. For tools and jewelry the Egyptians bartered for the precious myrrh resin as well as some myrrh saplings.

The Jews utilized myrrh in holy oil and medicines. Moses was instructed by God to use myrrh as one of the main ingredients in holy oil for anointing priests (Exodus 30:22–33). There are many other references to myrrh in the Bible, but the most striking is the section in the Song of Solomon that compares the joys of sexual love to myrrh (1:13 and 4:6). Myth tells us that the resin of this desert tree is an expression of the grief of Myrrha, a princess who was turned into the myrrh tree to escape the pain of incest.

Myrrh is one of several major medicinal tree resins found in global natural medicine. Frankincense is another prime example. The therapeutic values of these resins have been sadly neglected in modern countries. A closely related resin, gugulipid from the mukul myrrh tree, is a well-known Ayurvedic medicine, valued for the blood vessels and to lower cholesterol levels without the side effects of prescription drugs.

Health Benefits. Not surprisingly, myrrh has many medicinal virtues. Primarily, myrrh is considered cleansing and antiseptic: its cooling qualities are beneficial in sore throats, gum problems, mouth sores, and coughs. This resin is a good disinfectant often used to wash sores, cuts, and wounds. Incredibly enough, this most healing of substances enhances immune response, retards infections, and has antibiotic and antiviral properties.

First Aid. Healing for cuts, wounds, boils, and abrasions.

Primary Uses. Herbalists use myrrh to clear inflammation and infections and to promote tissue repair: especially gums, throat, stomach, and vagina; gingivitis, sore throat, laryngitis, menstrual problems, and coughs. It is used with other herbs for the common cold and expels cold mucus in the lungs: bronchitis. It combines well with echinacea or goldenseal. Frankincense and myrrh are commonly found in Oriental herbal formulas for muscular and arthritic pain. Myrrh, along with frankincense, is a major healing incense; to experience these aromas is healing for people who are depressed, grief-stricken, or coughing with damp phlegm.

Doses. Extracts or tablets, recommended doses; not a long-term remedy. For the average person, synergistic formulas with myrrh are adequate, ingesting 10 to 20 drops 2 to 3 times daily or as indicated.

Caution. Pregnant or lactating women, or those with kidney disease.

Note. The Ayurvedic myrrh, gum guggul, lowers cholesterol safely; see *Clinical Applications of Ayurvedic and Chinese Herbs*, by Kerry Bone (Warwick, Australia: Phytotherapy Press, 1996).

NETTLE, STINGING
Urtica dioica

HERB OF MANY USES

Stinging nettle is a global remedy found in Asia, Europe, and America and for hundreds of years has been used by every tradition where it grows, including American Indians, gypsies, homeopaths, Europeans of all countries, and the nineteenth-century Eclectics. Without doubt this medicinal plant can be called a power herb. It has the unusual distinction of being a source of fabric, a nutritious food, an herbal medicine, and a homeopathic remedy. The stings of the stinging nettle are real enough. Brush your arm against the furry leaves, and a sharp stinging sensation will irritate for a short time. Conventional doctors have missed the medicinal qualities of nettle, calling it an herb that has no pharmacological value when administered orally. This sad misunderstanding is all the more tragic when one considers that this herb, like dandelion and milk thistle, is of great value to busy modern people. Recent research into nettle leaf and root is demonstrating that the traditional herbalists were onto a valuable remedy.

Stinging nettle is not so common in New England, but there is a good patch in my garden, grown from seeds planted by the local herbalist, Helen Oshima. When I was a boy I had the good fortune to visit my aunt Mary in Midhurst, England. She owned a lovely country house in a rustic corner of Britain, an area rich with natural beauty as well as remnants from the past: Roman ruins, Druid stones, and Celtic mysteries. Much of my time was spent roaming the green hills where I first brushed up against the leaves of the green stinging nettle. Yes, nettle does sting, but not as sharp as a bee bite, and the discomfort passes quickly. On our walks we quickly learned to step around the thick clumps of the tall green nettle.

Nettle's place in literature is ensured; it is mentioned by Shakespeare, Chaucer, and other poets. Nettle is also a highly nutritious plant, probably more than any vegetable in the supermarket. For the thrifty Scots it was once a common food. Like dandelion and other wild greens, nettle can be a valuable addition to the white, pasty, modern diet because it provides excellent nourishment for the blood. It is best enjoyed in spring and early summer when the young shoots literally jump into the air and grow inches by the week. Gloves are used to harvest the plant, and cooking renders the prickly little leaf hairs harmless. Nettle can be enjoyed sautéed and steamed, alone or with other vegetables. I usually add a little seasoning, salt, pepper, and lemon, and it is as tasty as any other green. Don't underestimate its nutritive power; nettle is a superfood: it contains protein, iron, potassium, silica, chlorophyll, and one of the highest levels of calcium, magnesium, and zinc of any plant. This supergreen is one of the best for weak, anemic people and is certainly valuable for women who are thinking of getting pregnant.

The versatile nettle was once used to make cloth. As reported by Mrs. Grieve, the poet Thomas Campbell complained of the little attention paid to nettle in England:

"In Scotland, I have eaten nettles, I have slept on nettle sheets, and I have dined off of nettle table cloth. The young and tender nettle is an excellent potherb. The stalks of the old nettle are as good as flax for making cloth. I have heard my mother say that she thought nettle cloth more durable than any other species of linen."[23]

A useful plant indeed. But that is not all. The quick-growing nettle can be converted into sugars, starches, protein, ethyl alcohol, and methane gas and it is a very strengthening animal fodder. The root can be made into a dye and a medicine. Nettle can also produce paper, pudding, beer, and wine. Nettle beer was an old Scottish farmer remedy for gout and rheumatic pains. Nettle is one of the five herbs the Jews use to break the feast of Passover. In fact, the origin of the word goes back to an ancient Sanskrit word meaning to bind or sew, a reference to its use as a common fiber.

If you are a gardener and interested in nutritious foods, grow some nettle. You don't need a green thumb to be

23. Ibid., p. 575.

rewarded, and if you don't have the proverbial green thumb, don't despair. Greenness is within us all, and is simply a reflection of an inner warmth and caring for plants—which anybody can share. Also, once you have harvested the plant, look for the nettle pudding recipe in Mrs. Grieve's classic herb book, and you will share the same pleasure as the English writer Samuel Pepys. In his diary of February 1661, he writes, "We did eat some nettle paridge, which was very good."[24]

Health Benefits. Nettle's medicinal value exceeds its broad domestic uses. It is a versatile remedy, commonly used by modern homeopaths and botanical doctors. The plant has an ancient history. Dioscorides, the Greek doctor, used nettle tea for kidney and urinary problems and to expel stones. Nicholas Culpeper states that nettle is a fiery plant that rids the body of moistness and coldness, useful in opening the passages of the lungs, to cool inflammations of the mouth and throat, to expel gravel and stones.

Dr. James Compton Burnett, who used it for gout and allergic reactions, lauded stinging nettle. Dr. Compton Burnett, a famous turn-of-the-century London physician, served many of the aristocrats of his day. He introduced some important herbal remedies into homeopathy (and fathered a famous child, Ivy Compton Burnett, a novelist). Because homeopathic remedies are based on the principle of *like cures like*, stinging nettle lotion is a favorite for stings, mild burns, and rashes, its very effects when you rub up against it. I remember using it on my son Gabriel when he suffered from diaper rash; his cries stopped almost instantly. Homeopaths use the lotion and ointment as one of their major first-aid remedies,

24. Ibid., p. 577.

and for good reason. In my experience, it provides faster relief than aloe vera for minor burns. However, there is more to nettle than the leaf medicine. Recent studies indicate that nettle root is a healer for the kidney, bladder, and prostate.

First Aid. The homeopathic (*Urtica urens*) tincture and lotion is good for minor burns, itchy stings, and rashes. Internally, homeopaths recommend nettle in its homeopathic preparation for allergic reactions, particularly to shellfish and allergens.

Primary Uses. Modern herbalists are more than faithful to this ancient medicinal plant. The vegetable, extract, or tea are used to nourish the whole body. Herbalists use the leaf extract for skin inflammations, nosebleeds, hay fever, uterine bleeding, sinusitis, gout, and arthritis. Nettle root is now found in formulas for inflammation of the prostate gland and for urinary problems. Nettle tea is a hair tonic. Typically, nettle is used in synergistic formulas during hay fever season.

Health Promotion. Nettle leaf, often with other herbs, is a nutritional tonic that contains valuable nutrients and antioxidants for health promotion and disease prevention.

Dose. Capsules, extracts, and synergistic formulas, as recommended, but not for long-term use. A tea of the dried leaf is valued in Europe: 1 to 2 tablespoons in a cup of boiled water.

Complementary Remedies. Dandelion, burdock, red clover, and yellow dock. Nettle root is found in saw palmetto formulas for benign prostatic hyperplasia (BPH).

OLIVE OIL
and other vegetable oils
Olea europaea

MISSING NUTRIENTS

One of the signatures of ancient Greek civilization was the durable olive tree. The small gnarly evergreen olive tree still covers hills around the Mediterranean, particularly in Greece, Italy, and Spain, and today this region exports olive oil all over the globe. The dark purple fruit, the olive, is the source of one of the healthiest vegetable oils, a medicinal food by any standard.

Moses recognized the special value of olive oil. He exempted from military service the men who tended the olive trees. Egyptian pharaohs literally bathed in the oil. The Romans devoted many pages to extolling the wonders and virtues of the olive tree, and today one can still find Roman recipes that feature this oil. Olive oil is a staple in Italian cooking and is equally valued in other Mediterranean countries. Olive oil was regarded as an emblem of goodness and purity, and even today the leaves are a symbol of peace and goodwill.

Generally, fats have received a poor reputation in America, unfortunate because the healthy fats are not only essential for the life of the body but can prevent serious diseases. The culprit is not fats in general but the saturated fats and the hydrogenated fats, common in many processed oils and animal products. Olive oil is a monounsaturated fat that is easy for the body to assimilate, and, in fact, the monounsaturated fats of olive oil, unlike meat fats, processed oils, and margarine, promote good health, healthy arteries, and long life. People residing in regions where olive oil is a staple are known to have fewer heart attacks, arteriosclerosis, even cancer. For example, the people of the island of Crete eat more fat than most people but, paradoxically, have one of the lowest rates of heart disease and cancer in the world. Their main source of fat is the ubiquitous olive oil, pressed from trees growing all over their beautiful island. Dr. Andrew Weil also recommends canola oil for those who want an unflavored oil.

Olive oil has fundamental culinary and medicinal uses, and if that were not enough, the leaves contain antibacterial and antiviral properties. The oil is the basis of the healthy traditional Italian cuisine, which is founded on power herbs and foods: garlic, olive oil, green vegetables, green herbs like basil, as well as rice, pasta, and moderate amounts of meat and fish.

The best olive oil is cold pressed, not prepared with heat or chemicals, and best of all is the virgin first pressed. Olive oil should, of course, have a prime place in the kitchen, but it is also a power remedy in its own right. If necessary, it can be ingested in small amounts for overall health and the cardiovascular system. Externally, it is good for the skin and hair.

Other plants that contain healthful oils include the primrose flower, flaxseed, pumpkin seed, and borage seed. Flaxseed, for example, is an excellent source of omega-3 fatty acids, an essential fatty acid often lacking in modern diet. Modern diet has excess saturated fats and is now deficient in essential fatty acids, particularly omega-3, essential for the health of the nerves, heart, connective tissue, and muscles. Prostaglandins, partially formed from these fatty acids, moderate inflammations in the body. Essential fatty acids are now valued in the treatment of arthritis, diseases of the nervous system, constipation, and bowel disorders.

Unfortunately, the American food industry floods the

market with unhealthy saturated and hydrogenated fats that clog the body like sludge. Essential fatty acids have almost been eliminated from the food sources, replaced by trans fatty acids and partially hydrogenated oils (a favorite of the food industry) that are difficult for the body to break apart and utilize. Margarine is the ultimate representation of a hydrogenated fat substance. Once the darling of the food industry, margarine does not spoil easily, for obvious reasons—the fatty acid chains are glued together. No wonder the body cannot assimilate these "wonder" foods. Contrary to the current phobia of fats, fats are not only good for us, they are absolutely essential—that is, the good, unsaturated fats like cold-pressed olive, canola, and sunflower oil. Since these fatty acids are so important in the body, it is remarkable that the majority of Americans (up to 80 percent) are deficient in them.

Many people know that hydrogenated fats, as found in "foods" like margarine, lard, and "cooked" oils, are not healthy for the human body. Most people do not know, however, about the harmful effects of *trans fatty* acids, the by-product of the commercially processed polyunsaturated vegetable oils. Unrefined polyunsaturated oils contain healthful fatty acids, but once exposed to high heat and hydrogenation in the process of "refinement," they are transformed into harmful compounds. The FDA has not mandated the disclosure of trans fatty acids in commercial oils, but the label *hydrogenated* is a telltale warning. Dr. Donald Rudin, who has researched the importance of essential fatty acids, reports that studies have revealed countless dangers of trans fatty acids. They increase the formation of free radicals, lower beneficial HDL cholesterol, diminish the quality of breast milk, decrease levels of testosterone, alter cell membranes, and block utilization of essential fatty acids.

Olive oil is probably the best all-around kitchen oil and is an essential staple for modern people. Other vegetable oils particularly rich in essential fatty acids (especially omega-3) are important food supplements for a limited period of time for particular health problems. The main health benefits of the major plant oils are listed hereafter, but it should not be forgotten that the oils in fish, particularly cold-water fish, are also beneficial for overall health. For optimum functioning of the healthy fats it is necessary to reduce, or even avoid, excess meat fats, overly cooked fats, and hydrogenated oils.

Evening Primrose Oil (Oenothera biennis) is a modern food supplement rich in essential fatty acids, particularly gamma-linolenic acid (GLA). This oil is beneficial for breast tenderness and PMS and is valued as an overall health promoter. It can lower cholesterol, soothe dry irritated skin, benefit the heart, and lower blood pressure. Capsules (250 milligrams) can be taken up to 3 times a day for a specific period, as recommended.

Flaxseeds are especially high in omega-3 fatty acids and lignans, both compounds with health benefits for many conditions, including arthritis, constipation, diseases of the nervous system, cancer, high cholesterol, and inflammatory skin problems. Ground flaxseeds can be added to other foods like breads or porridges. Flaxseed oil is also valued as a supplement, but for the short term, and only bona fide expeller-pressed oil of high quality. High-heat processing and chemicals will destroy the health benefits of this remarkable healing substance.

Olive oil can be used daily in cooking and salad dressings, or taken as a food supplement (1 to 2 teaspoons once or twice daily). This beneficent oil has multiple uses.

1. A mild and safe laxative (1 to 2 ounces daily for a few days)
2. Stimulates production of bile in the liver
3. Soothes dry skin, itching, and insect bites
4. Reduces "bad" cholesterol in the blood and is good for the heart and cardiovascular system
5. Internally and externally, improves the beauty of the hair and skin
6. May inhibit cancer and aging

In addition, olive leaf extract in capsules can be taken to boost the immune system and inhibit the growth of harmful fungi, viruses, and bacteria.

Note. The best source of all oils are those not exposed to high heat and chemicals, most often found in quality health food stores. Vegetable oils produced with high heat or chemicals, even when labeled cold pressed, can contain harmful molecules. Some manufacturers sacrifice quality for quantity. Shop carefully, read labels, and ask questions.

Caution. Pregnant women should not use excessive amounts of vegetable oils as a supplement because of the laxative and uterine effect.

PAU D'ARCO
Tabebuia impetiginosa
Also called lapacho and taheebo

RAIN FOREST MEDICINE
The huge Amazon basin is filled with abundant plant life, including many useful medicines. In North America probably the best known of these is pau d'arco. A beautiful and abundant tree, pau d'arco is a gift to us from the great jungles of Brazil, Argentina, Paraguay, and Peru. This hardy tree would not survive in the damp, microbe-rich jungle without potent phytochemicals that resist fungi, viruses, and bacteria. The Inca Indians of Peru, who called pau d'arco the divine tree, considered it a sacred plant. Rain forest tribes have been familiar with this potent medicinal tree for hundreds of years, and it is still extraordinarily popular for jungle skin diseases: rashes, eczema, fungal infections, and unspecified lumps. Similar species are used in Asia for medicinal purposes. The medicine is extracted from the inner bark of the tree, and key constituents include lapachol and beta-lapachon, both of which possess antifungal and possible antitumor properties.

In the jungles of South America, this herbal medicine has a legendary reputation as a cure-all. I will be mindful of the exaggeration and bring its practical uses into focus. Also called lapacho, pau d'arco is recognized in herbal medicine as a profound cleanser of the blood and skin, particularly of fungi and other pernicious microbes. It has antibiotic and antiviral properties, and many claim pau d'arco is a cure for cancer. While it might be useful in a comprehensive program, there is no evidence that this herb is a magic bullet for cancer. In relation to its treatment for cancer, the herb was studied by the American Cancer Society at the National Institutes of Health, but the whole herb was never tested. In the cancer testing they used highly purified individual constituents (napthaquinones) and determined that in vitro these have no antitumor activity—a conclusion that virtually closed the book on further research, at least in this country. In South America pau d'arco remains one of the most popular herbs to assist in treatment of patients with cancer and other chronic diseases.

First Aid. Used for fungal and skin problems.

Primary Uses. In the jungle pau d'arco is used to treat parasites and funguses, as well as numerous skin problems, tumors, ulcers, and wounds. It is said to be a tonic for the liver and can be used by people undergoing chemotherapy. This herb may find wider use for chronic skin problems like eczema and for autoimmune diseases. It is used for all fungus problems, internal infestations (candida) as well as those on the skin (athlete's foot). With the consultation of a physician this herb is prescribed as an adjunct treatment for adult-onset diabetes, and it may yet prove helpful for cancer patients. Herbalists also commonly use this versatile plant for colds, flu, sore throats, viral infections, herpes, and rashes.

Health Promotion. One can use pau d'arco periodically (a tea for several weeks), especially for those undergoing high stress and health transition. It can be used for those recovering from long-term illness (with the approval of a doctor) and for those who have been sick in the tropics.

Doses. In tablets, capsules, and extracts; extract 10 to 20 drops 2 to 3 times daily or as directed by a professional. Pau d'arco is often prepared as a tea, 2 to 3 teaspoons simmered in a pint of water for 15 to 20 minutes (do not overboil);

standardized extracts or capsules provide the guaranteed constituents. Pau d'arco is also favored in synergistic extract formulas as a disease preventative. Some sources of this plant medicine are said to be questionable, so buy the bark from a reputable source. Extracts from quality companies are assayed for reliability.

Cautions. This is a safe herb when taken according to instructions, but a few cases of indigestion have been reported. Avoid during pregnancy or lactation.

Complementary Remedies. Chaparral, echinacea, goldenseal, and cat's claw (*Uncaria tomentosa*).

PEPPERMINT AND OTHER MINTS
Mentha piperita

HAPPY MINT

The mints—spearmint, water mint, and peppermint—have been common household remedies for centuries. Universal medicines, they can be found in most healing traditions. Peppermint, the most important medicinal mint, is a complex hybrid of mints with a very intricate genetic composition. Strangely enough, it was not recognized as a distinct species of mint until the great botanist John Ray wrote about it in 1696. The major medicinal component of peppermint is menthol, which exists in the volatile oil of the plant. Without any doubt, peppermint is a power herb of remarkable versatility and is much recommended for home use.

Greek mythology tells us that Pluto, god of the underworld, introduced mints to the earth after he fell in love with a beautiful nymph, Minthe. His affair enraged his wife,

Persephone, who changed poor Minthe into an herb. The grief-stricken Pluto could not undo the damage and offered Minthe her unforgettable aroma, which would soothe people for centuries to come. In Roman times Pliny mentions that mints were much used in the kitchen and apothecary. Egyptians also fancied mint, and in the oldest medical text, the Ebers Papyrus, mint is recognized as a calmative for the stomach. Even the Bible can't resist mentioning this most favorite of herbs. In ancient Palestine mint was accepted as a payment of taxes. In Luke (11:39) Jesus scolds the Pharisees: "You pay tithes of mint and rue . . . but have no care for justice and the love of God."

Health Benefits. There is hardly a famous herbalist through history who has not praised peppermint, and today modern research has confirmed that peppermint oil has germicidal and antispasmodic properties. In the nineteenth century the Eclectics recognized the analgesic and decongestant properties of peppermint, accounting for its continued popularity in modern ointments and creams, including Solarcaine, Ben-Gay, and Vicks VapoRub. Most of the world's nations have used mints, often for digestion, coughs, colds, and intestinal woes, but peppermint is more than a simple home remedy. Menthol, the most active ingredient in peppermint, is an antispasmodic and is therefore useful for problems of intestinal or stomach cramping. Peppermint helps to prevent ulcers and to stimulate bile secretion, and the menthol vapors are well known for their ability to open the sinuses and relieve congestion of the nose or lungs. A popular remedy for the common cold, the essential oil of peppermint even has antiviral and antibacterial properties. Peppermint is also a folk remedy for menstrual cramps and morning sickness. Herbalists consider peppermint warming and dispersing, soothing for the stomach, and beneficial for the lungs, the intestine, and the liver and gallbladder.

First Aid. Peppermint oil has analgesic properties, and a few drops can be rubbed on the temple to relieve a headache. A strong cup of peppermint tea is recommended for headaches, and, in fact, for many minor pains and aches.

Primary Uses. Colds, sinus problems, headaches; soothes and calms the stomach, nausea, and vomiting; intestinal gas and irritable bowels; relaxes the muscles; stimulates the flow of bile. For irritable bowels seek professional advice—only coated pills of peppermint are used for bowel problems to bypass stomach acids. The tea is valuable for those with gallbladder problems.

Doses. A tea made from the leaves, often in combination with herbs like chamomile. Extract, tablets, and capsules are available, as well as synergistic formulas. Peppermint is not an herb to take every day for a long time, but occasionally when needed, and best in strong herbal teas.

Caution. Considered a safe herbal tea, but use weak potions for the younger ones. For those with liver or gallbladder problems, seek medical advice.

POWER FOODS
Oats, tomato, soybean, greens, onions, and grapes

MEDICINAL GEMS, DAILY FOOD
In a book on power herbs one cannot overlook the therapeutic value of certain foods, a few of which could be classi-

fied as power herbs in their own right. Daily foods and nutrition are a fundamental part of health and healing, and most natural foods have nourishing, if not medicinal, qualities. For centuries a major part of traditional medical systems—Oriental, East Indian, and tribal—has been food. The traditional Oriental physician will often first prescribe dietary (often along with lifestyle changes like exercises) as his first defense against disease.

In Oriental medicine there is a whole branch that has to do with utilizing foods as medicine, and all foods are classified according to their energetic action and nutritional benefits. Changes in diet will often be first prescribed for many common health problems, even conditions such as high blood pressure and migraine headaches. If the food and common-sense therapy do not work, then the doctor will advise medicinal herbs, more potent than the foods. The potent drugs, the major armory of current Western medicine, are the last line of defense and traditionally are used only when lifestyle changes, diet, and herbs do not work.

Some foods are such useful medicines that they are part of the herbal medicine. These, like garlic, are more potent than your typical daily food and are commonly used for specific disease problems. A few of these have been included as power herbs, most notably the inimitable duo of ginger and garlic. Common daily foods, however, are very nourishing and healing and should be respected for their actions and benefit to the human body.

For the purposes of this book, I will not discuss the nutritional benefits of many important foods, including meats, grains (with the exception of oats), and others, but will focus on a select group that have come into prominence recently.

Modern research is validating what Granny said all those years: many foods are not only healthful but can prevent disease. Recent research has been uncovering a wealth of constituents in common foods that have specific medicinal properties.

POWER FOODS: A SAMPLING

Oats. A power medicine in its own right. The *extract of oat* is a specific herbal medicine for strengthening the body and nervous system, particularly for recovering alcoholics and drug addicts and for exhaustion. The oat grain is also a good everyday preventative medicine for everyone, an extraordinary food with few comparisons. Oats are a rich source of fiber, nutrients, and carbohydrates; they are warming, calming, and strengthening, one of the perfect foods for people living in cold climates. They are healthy for the whole digestive system, and a regular use of oats is known to help prevent digestive disorders, particularly of the intestines.

Greens. Such an important class of medicinal foods that they have their own entry; see *Greens*.

Tomatoes. This much-loved vegetable is the number-one source of lycopene, the pigment that makes tomatoes red. Lycopene is another super antioxidant that protects the body from disease. Ingestion of lycopene is said to inhibit such diseases as prostate cancer. In countries where tomatoes are commonly consumed, prostrate cancer is up to 40 percent less common. Of course, other factors must be taken into account: other foods and lifestyle. Lycopene, most fortunately, is not destroyed by heat. Watermelon, red cabbage, and red grapefruit also contain lycopene.

Onions. An ancient medicinal food much respected by

Egyptians, Romans, Indians, and Orientals. Onions have now been "discovered" by modern medicine! Onions lower blood pressure and protect the body from disease agents. For example, they contain quercetin, a formidable antioxidant with anticancer, antifungal, and antibacterial properties. They also thin the blood and help to prevent blood clotting. A Dutch study revealed that those who ate one-half an onion a day reduced the incidence of stomach cancer by one-half (see *The Food Pharmacy*, by Jean Carper). Those eating antioxidant-rich foods like kale, onion, garlic, apples, and broccoli are less likely to suffer heart attacks.

Grapes. Red wine and red grape juice are happily loaded with the antioxidants known as flavonoids and phenols. Grapes and wine made from red grapes help to thin the blood, lower cholesterol, and boost immunity. Amazingly enough, they also fight allergies and inhibit cancer. *Grape seed extract* is a potent remedy in its own right.

Soybeans. Known to inhibit cancer, particularly of the breast, ovaries, and prostate, soybeans contain isoflavones, particularly genistein. Research now indicates that genistein and other isoflavones can protect the body from carcinogens. This valuable food, a favorite of Asian cooks and physicians, also reduces blood cholesterol and the incidence of hot flashes. Soybeans are commonly converted into soy milk, tofu, and soy flour. Soybean oil and soy sauce do not contain the healing compound genistein. Interesting that the traditional diet of Orientals is loaded with healthful power foods: fresh greens, soy products, green herbs, onions, carrots, and garlic. Sad to think that many Orientals are now enticed by the modern American junk food diet: greasy hamburgers and chips, salty foods, an overload of saturated fats, and a paucity of fresh greens and fiber foods.

Beets. The humble beet, the main ingredient of the famous Russian soup borscht, could be a power herb in its own right. For centuries herbalists have recognized that beets are a superior healing vegetable. Beets contain a host of nutritious and healing antioxidants, particularly therapeutic for the liver, blood, and immune system. Beet juice is one of the most healing juices for chronic degenerative illness, including cancer and AIDS, and beet extract is often found in herbal blood-cleansing formulas.

RED CLOVER
Trifolium pratense

CONTROVERSIAL FIELD HERB
The luckiest cows in the world are those from Vermont. Each day they chomp on the state flower, red clover, a nourishing herb that is adorned by rose and pink flower heads. Red clover is somewhat controversial because of its association with several traditional formulas for treating cancer. While these formulas might not cure cancer, there is good reason to say they could help cancer patients in their healing passage. The fact remains, however, that this herb of the fields is far more than a curiosity. Herbal tradition suggests that it is a potent healer of the whole body, but particularly the lungs, skin, and liver. Modern research is beginning to verify the true therapeutic value of this ancient medicine.

Red clover, one of the largest of the various clover species, is an herb that has been associated with good fortune. Visitors traveling through lands where spirits might lurk often carried a sprig, and the famous mutation, the four-leaf clover, is still considered a sign of good luck. American Indians had many uses for this humble herb, which can grow as high as 3 feet, including eating the green as a spring vegetable. Externally they used it for ulcers, burns, and lumps, and in time red clover passed into white folk medicine and herbalism. The eminent Eclectic physician Dr. Harvey W. Felter valued red clover for its general health benefits but found it particularly nourishing for cancer and other chronic diseases, skin problems, and coughing.

Health Benefits. The flower heads are the principal source of the herbal medicine. Modern herbalists consider red clover a major alterative and blood purifier, a plant that can alter disease predisposition—as well as a cough medicine and antispasmodic. Historically it has been extensively used for lumps, eczema, and rashes. Red clover is rich in nutrients, particularly minerals like calcium, magnesium, and potassium. Modern research has yet to confirm its use for tumors, but it is now said that two constituents, genistein and biochanin A, have antitumor properties. Modern research is still exploring a group of compounds called isoflavones, of which genistein and biochanin A are the most interesting from a therapeutic point of view. Soybeans, another good source of genistein, are now believed to inhibit the formation of cancer. James A. Duke, a modern authority on medicinal plants, urges that red clover warrants further examination.

First Aid. Flower head poultice is applied to burns, rashes, and itches.

Primary Uses. Herbalists value this herb for coughs, externally to relieve psoriasis and eczema, and for bronchitis and whooping cough. Overall it is considered a valuable "blood purifier," thus good for disease prevention and overall health.

Health Promotion. This herb is good for health promotion and possibly cancer prevention. Red clover is a notable herbal medicine for its nourishing and healing qualities.

Doses. Extract or capsules 2 to 3 times daily in recommended doses. The tea is highly recommended, as well as synergistic formulas.

Caution. Those on blood thinners should avoid this herb, as well as pregnant women.

Complementary Remedies. In skin problems: red clover is often combined with nettle and yellow dock, a very healing trio. In adjunct therapy for cancer this herb has been used with nettle leaf, pau d'arco, burdock, chaparral, barberry, and other herbs.

RED RASPBERRY
Rubus idaeus

FEMALE REMEDY

Raspberry leaves have an ancient history in Europe and other parts of our planet. In fact, this is another global medicine, appreciated by the Europeans, Chinese, Greeks, Egyptians, and many other people. Red raspberry, a member of the rose family, is native to England, where it thrives along hedges and roadsides. Today raspberry is cultivated all over the planet. The much-loved fruit is enjoyed by many and in creative kitchens is converted into jellies, jams, vinegar, and wines. Because of its tannins, raspberry is a well-known astringent, soothing for sore throats and diarrhea. One of the most common herbal teas, raspberry is also a common female remedy.

Raspberry leaves, interestingly enough, are very high in nutrients, especially vitamin C, iron, manganese, and niacin. The leaves contain more manganese than most vegetables or fruits. The ancients were really onto something when they respected the humble leaves of this common bush. Manganese promotes healthy nerves and the immune system, is required for normal bone growth and to prevent anemia, and is also needed to utilize thiamin and vitamin E. Furthermore, manganese, along with B vitamins, helps to induce a feeling of well-being, aids in the formation of mother's milk, and is necessary for protein and fat metabolism.

The raspberry fruit is also a medicine, used as a nutritive and blood tonic in European and other herbal systems. Called *Fu pen zi* in Chinese herbalism, the fruit is a mild tonic for kidneys, particularly to prevent night urination, and a gentle stimulant for the kidney yang, which is the force behind the sex drive.

Health Benefits. Raspberry leaf is one of the major women's remedies, but particularly for those in childbearing years. Taken regularly, raspberry is said to strengthen and tone the womb and ease labor pains. It can also be used by anyone for diarrhea, sore throats, and bleeding gums. For centuries raspberry was one of the major herbal remedies of the midwife, who not too long ago was also an herbalist. She would recommend the tea during the last two months of pregnancy and after the birth to support the overall health. Today this herb is also used for menstrual cramping, often in synergistic formulas. Scientific studies have revealed that raspberry contains chemicals that benefit the uterus, and the tannins in the plant are responsible for its astringent qualities. Raspberry could be an adjunct treatment for some kinds of cancer because of antioxidants, flavonoids, and tannins found in the leaves. In *The Green Pharmacy*, Dr. James A. Duke, one of America's experts about medicinal plants, recommends raspberry for its traditional healing benefits.[25]

First Aid. Raspberry is a common remedy for mild sore throats and gum problems and is used for gargling.

Primary Uses. Bleeding and spongy gums, diarrhea, and sore throat; uterine tonic, cramping, and morning sickness. Under the guidance of a professional this herb can be used during the last trimester. Midwife herbalists value this herb for a wide range of women's problems, particularly to assist in easing the labor and to enrich and cleanse the milk of a nursing mother.

Health Promotion. A mild but important tonic for women, this herb also is valuable for children and men; and quite clearly a valuable tea for every household.

Dose. 1 cup of tea 2 to 3 times daily; extract or in synergistic formulas. This plant is a safe natural medicine.

Complementary Remedies. Blue cohosh, schisandra, motherwort, and vitex. Blackberry leaves are often used in conjunction with red raspberry.

25. James A. Duke, *The Green Pharmacy* (New York: St. Martin's, 1998), p. 396.

REHMANNIA
Rehmannia glutinosa
Di-huang

LONGEVITY HERB

Rehmannia is another great Oriental herb that is not yet well known in America. This healing plant not only is very common in Oriental medicine and has been valued for hundreds of years, but it can help conditions that are endemic in the hectic modern world. Rehmannia, prepared from the root, is one of the best remedies for symptoms resulting from excess stress, nervousness, overwork, anxiety, and aging. With the usual complexity of Chinese herbalism, rehmannia is made in three forms: dried, fresh, and prepared. While the action of these preparations is somewhat similar, most important here is the prepared herbal medicine *Shu-di-huang.* The dried roots are steamed to a black color, then dried again, a process that refines the medicinal action of this excellent healer. Often used in complex multitiered herbal formulas, rehmannia is prescribed for a variety of conditions related to overwork of organs and the nervous system.

Rehmannia has a long history of use in the Far East. One of the first recorded uses of the prepared root occurred during the Song dynasty (1061 A.D.) in the *Tu Jing Ben Cao,* by Su Song. The deepest healing benefits of this plant were discovered by ancient herbalists who first washed the root in wine, steamed it on a willow frame in a porcelain vessel, then dried, resteamed, and redried it nine times until the root attained a shiny black color. *Di-huang,* meaning yellow earth, remains to this day one of the major Oriental herbs, found in numerous clinics and pharmacies around the globe.

Health Benefits. Rehmannia has several important healing actions. Oriental herbalists consider rehmannia one of their major restorative herbs because it treats a symptom picture called liver blood and kidney yin deficiency. This picture, very relevant for modern people, can result in the following symptoms: loss of stamina, palpitations, restlessness, fatigue, muscle aches, diabetes, deafness, vertigo, general malaise, scanty menses, ringing in the ears, night sweats, low back pain, and poor sleep. From a Western point of view this remedy benefits the liver, blood, and nervous system, and is helpful in a variety of conditions, including arthritis, anxiety, fatigue, menstrual problems, hypertension, and hepatitis. Modern Chinese studies have revealed some important properties: it appears to lower blood pressure, cholesterol, and blood sugar levels.

Primary Uses. Poor stamina, excess stress syndromes, nervousness, and a variety of symptoms and conditions already listed. In Chinese medicine rehmannia is a main herb to nourish what is called the kidney essence, the very root of health.

Health Promotion. Definitely a health-promoting herbal medicine, rehmannia and its complementary herbs deserve greater recognition in the West.

Doses. This herb can be found in all pharmacies that sell crude Oriental herbs, in Oriental patent herb formulas, and in some synergistic herbal formulas manufactured in the West. Typical dose of a liquid extract: 20 to 30 drops 2 times a day for several weeks, or as recommended.

Rehmannia is the principal herb in several classic herbal formulas. For example, the superb "Six-ingredient pill with rehmannia" is one that can be purchased in America as a prepared medicine, usually pills or capsules. The key function of this famous formula is to tone and restore the kidney and liver yin depletion, symptoms of aggravated stress such as night sweating, palpitations, dizziness, anxiousness, and low back pain. The elegance of an Oriental herbal formula can be admired in the multitiered structure, consisting of two groups of three herbs each. In the first group of herbs rehmannia is the chief or "kingly" herb; the three secondary or deputy herbs support the liver and the metabolism, and act in various physiological ways as assistants to the first, balancing and enhancing the effects of the whole formula. This, and similar formulas, is said to "nourish the essence and support the spirit," in other words prolong life, and is a tonic to virtually every function and organ of the body. Both men and women benefit from rehmannia.

Complementary Remedies. The power herbs he shou wu, astragalus, dong quai, and ligustrum.

REISHI MUSHROOM
Ganoderma lucidum
Ling zhi cao

MUSHROOM OF LONGEVITY

A premier remedy in Oriental medicine, reishi (the Japanese name) is one of several important medicinal mushrooms. Oriental herbalists have utilized mushroom medicines for many centuries, along with those in Russia, Latvia, and many eastern European countries. The ancient Taoist priests of China considered reishi an elixir of immortality, also calling it the herb of spiritual potency. Reishi, however, is not a culinary herb; it is a fibrous shelf mushroom.

Mushrooms, often looked at with suspicion in the West (particularly England and America), are highly valued as a food and medicine in Asia. It is curious that even in the Western herbal tradition the therapeutic benefits of mushrooms have been largely overlooked. This neglect may have to do with the fact that Western people have harbored a lingering fear of the unknown in nature—mushrooms being a potent symbol of wild nature. It is true that there are a few species of poisonous mushrooms, but these are relatively easy to identify and make up a very small proportion of the mushroom population. Reishi, a large reddish shelf mushroom, is easy to identify and so distinctive and beautiful that it is made into art objects and decorations. Like many herbs (St. John's wort is also a good example), reishi has been used in folk traditions to protect against bad luck and evil spirits. We are now discovering that these herbs are truly healing for the spirit or essence of a person, perhaps accounting for their durable if fanciful reputations in folk medicine.

Italians, Russians, Chinese, and many other people have a long tradition of enjoying wild mushrooms. Every summer Italians begin an exodus to secret spots to find their favorite culinary mushrooms. In fact, mushrooms like *Boletus edulis* are considered a superb delicacy. In Oriental herbalism, many wild mushrooms are also considered excellent healing foods. Nonetheless, people should not venture into the woods to hunt for mushrooms without expert guidance. Traditionally Granny or the local herbalist was the initial guide. In America there are now mushroom clubs that offer expertise, such as the mycology club of Boston with whom I enjoy forays in the local woods. Learning the edible mushrooms is relatively easy, and the hunt, as well as the subsequent feasts, truly a delight.

Health Benefits. The healing properties of mushrooms are numerous, and the species of mushrooms that are used as medicines are more than a handful. Reishi, or *ling zhi*, is a premier mushroom in Oriental herbal medicine, but there are several important species that are gaining respect in the West. Most recognizable to Americans is the popular culinary shiitake, a mushroom that is made into a modern medicine in Japan. Shiitake boosts the immune systems of people undergoing chemotherapy and is valued as a remedy for blood pressure and high cholesterol. Another mushroom, hen of the woods (*Grifola frondalosa*), can be found in American woods. Hen of the woods shows promise as a medicine for breast cancer patients, not as a cure but an adjunct treatment. Currently, there is growing interest in the healing benefit of all these mushrooms.

A major adaptogen, reishi is also considered an herb of spiritual potency. Just as mushrooms help to recycle life in the forest, so can the medicine transform waste and negativity in the body. In the Orient reishi is said to nourish the blood and energy and to strengthen the major organs, especially the liver and heart. It also soothes and calms the spirit. Scientific research, mostly conducted in the Orient, indicates numerous medicinal actions, including antitumor, immune modulating, and antiviral activity, as well as some distinct nutritional properties. Constituents have been found that support the heart and relieve coughing, asthma, and shortness of breath. In fact, reishi's broad health benefits are due to a complex synergy of constituents, including polysaccharides, which stimulate the immune function, triterpene acids, which protect the liver and reduce hypertension, and an alkaloid that benefits the heart. On reflection it is somewhat astonishing that most of the traditional Oriental uses have been supported by recent research, but in the West reishi's clinical potential has yet to be fully examined or tested.

Primary Uses. Herbalists use this herb alone and in formulas for weakened conditions, recovery from debilitating disease and surgery, fatigue, chronic coughs and asthma, digestive weakness, headaches, insomnia, palpitations, nervousness, and chemical detoxification. Reishi also detoxifies the effects of poisonous mushrooms (after medical assistance) and is valued in cases of immune deficiency, radiation poisoning, adrenal insufficiency, menopause, ulcer, and hyperlipidemia.

Health Promotion. Quite clearly reishi promotes good health.

Doses. Capsules, tablets, and liquid extracts, as directed, often 2 to 3 times daily for several weeks. Decoctions are prepared from whole mushroom. Reishi is found in synergistic formulas for the vital energy and immune system, often with other mushrooms or herbs.

Complementary Remedies. Shiitake is a delicious medicinal mushroom that can be easily added to vegetable and meat dishes. In Oriental medicine, all mushrooms are considered healthful, even the common supermarket variety, but a few species like reishi, maitake (hen of the woods), and shiitake are especially valuable. Reishi is well complemented by American ginseng, St. John's wort, and gotu kola.

Caution. Rare digestive symptoms from long-term use; consult a physician for those on blood thinners and for those pregnant or lactating.

Note. I recommend *Medicinal Mushrooms*, by the herbalist Christopher Hobbs.

ROSEMARY
Rosmarinus officinalis

QUEEN OF THE GARDEN HERBS

Rosemary, a small evergreen shrub, thrives on the sunny, rocky hills of southern France. In fact it can be found all around the Mediterranean, especially near the sea. Its botanical name means dew of the sea. Nowadays, rosemary is raised all over the planet, planted in gardens in the summer or on window ledges. This hardy perennial can even be found growing wild in the Sahara desert.

Rosemary bears humble but beautiful little blue flowers. As with most famous herbs, stories and legends surround this plant. There is even one to explain the blue of the flower. The Virgin Mary, forced to escape the arrest of Herod's soldiers, fled into the desert carrying the Christ Child. One night as they lay down to rest, Mary laid her blue cloak onto a rosemary bush bearing white flowers. The next morning the flowers had turned to the color of her cloak, and the plant was called Rose of Mary.

During the early Middle Ages, Charlemagne, the great king of France, ordered that rosemary be cultivated on the imperial farms. The superb monastery gardens of those times also prized the plant. Rosemary, another good-luck plant, is said to protect against witchcraft and evil spirits. Interestingly enough, the leaves and twigs have a long history of protecting against disease and plague. Rosemary was commonly burned in hospitals and towns during plagues. We now know that the plant has germicide properties.

This versatile herb has many roles in the life of people. It is a much-loved kitchen herb, added to soups, lamb dishes, stews, and bread. The dried twigs, like cedar shavings, repel insects and can be placed in drawers and cupboards. Rosemary, most famous for its lively aroma, was one of the first essential oils to be manufactured. Around 1330, Raymundus Lullus produced the oil by vaporization and condensation, and from that time this oil entered the pantheon of great therapeutic aromatic essences, valued as an ingredient in soaps, bath oils, colognes, and cosmetics. Rosemary is one of the queens of aromatherapy, a distinct branch of herbal medicine that heals with the aromas of plants. In the seventeenth century, Nicholas Culpeper said that rosemary helps "cold diseases of the head and brain, as the giddiness and swimmings therein, drowsiness or dullness . . . weak memory, and quickens the senses."[26]

Health Benefits. Rosemary presents us with a classic case of a traditional herb finding modern meaning because of recent scientific research, uncovering that the intuitions and experience of the traditional herbalists were right on target much of the time. Recent studies have revealed that rosemary does indeed improve thought processes by stimulating the action of brain neurotransmitters. This herb contains powerful antioxidants, including rosmarinic acid, which account for some of its medicinal powers. It also contains antibiotic properties.

Subtler, however, are the related aromatic healing powers of rosemary, valued by the Greeks, Arabs, French, and many other peoples. This plant has a very distinct and pungent aroma. It penetrates but does not overwhelm the nostrils and brain. Traditionally, all cultures where this plant lives recognize that its scent is enlivening and awakening. It calls us to

26. Culpeper, *Culpeper's Complete Herbal.*

remember. Oriental medicine calls this aroma yang: clear, active, strong, and resonant. Because of its association with memory, rosemary is connected to the two primary cycles of life, birth and death, and it often signifies the fidelity of two lovers. It has played a common role in Christian ceremonies, particularly the wedding and funeral. The bride commonly wore rosemary twigs in a wreath, and at the end of life the grave was sprinkled with the dried leaves. Robert Herrick, the English poet, wrote: "Grow for two ends, matters not at all / be it for my bridal or my burial." And of course there is the famous line in Shakespeare where the grieving Ophelia, soon to drown herself, laments Hamlet's confusion: "There's rosemary, that for remembrance: pray you, love, remember."

In herbalism, rosemary is considered a warming, stimulating herb that awakens the brain and nervous system and promotes healing and happiness. Increasing evidence indicates that rosemary can indeed improve the memory, even proving helpful for patients suffering from Alzheimer's disease. In his recent book *The Green Pharmacy*, Dr. James A. Duke says that rosemary contains several compounds that prevent the breakdown of acetylcholine, an important neurotransmitter in the brain.[27] One is left with a question: How did all those many generations of herbalists, poets, and country folk know and maintain the tradition that rosemary was beneficial for memory and the brain?

First Aid. Rosemary bath salts or essential oil can be used in baths for people who are recovering from accidents, exhaustion, stress, and trauma.

Primary Uses. Aromatherapists, who know the medicinal

27. Duke, *The Green Pharmacy*, pp. 47–48.

value of essential oils better than most, use rosemary oil in massage lotions and baths and for inhaling, for activating the mind and memory, and for its general enlivening qualities. It is also valued for head colds, drowsiness, and lethargy. Herbalists use the tea and extract for similar purposes, as well as to stimulate the liver and gallbladder, for stomachaches, to stimulate the hair and scalp, and to activate the immune system. Rosemary is a cold remedy, especially for "damp" chilly colds, and one of the best oils for massage and baths.

Doses. An essential oil, a tea, and a tincture—also found in synergistic herbal formulas for the brain, memory, and digestive system.

Caution. No one should ingest the essential oil, especially not pregnant or lactating women.

Complementary Remedies. Oil of lavender, another remarkable aromatic remedy, is also therapeutic for the nervous system.

ST. JOHN'S WORT
Hypericum perforatum

HERBAL SUPERSTAR

St. John's wort, a common weed, is often found in abandoned fields and along roadsides. It is a humble herb, often a foot or two high, decorated by small yellow flowers that begin to bloom in early summer, in fact around the time of the summer solstice. When the stem is broken, the plant expresses a reddish juice, a signature of its medicinal powers, specifically in the healing of wounds. The plant is in full flower by St. John's Day, June 24, the day the saint was beheaded. *Herba Sancti Ioannis*, the herb of St. John, became known as St. John's wort. *Wort* is a medieval word for *plant*. The whole plant can be used to make an extract or tea, but the flowers and buds are considered the cream of the plant.

Through time St. John's wort has been considered a magical plant that could ward off evil spirits and promote good luck. In modern times we automatically deride these ancient "superstitions"—and some of them do deserve skepticism—but in the case of this herb, research is bearing out many of the traditional claims. St. John's wort is a medicinal storehouse that can indeed bring good fortune and health into people's lives. Ironically, this herb has recently received some astonishing publicity due to scientific research and is now found even in most pharmacies across our nation.

St. John's wort has been valued by many cultures for thousands of years. The Greek physician Dioscorides knew of its value as a wound healer; so did the medieval monks and women healers. The sixteenth-century master herbalist John Gerard wrote that it is "a most precious remedie for deep wounds and those that are through the bodie or any wound made with a venomed weapon." Many of these traditional healers recognized that this plant helped people who were unhappy or emotionally upset.

The founder of homeopathy, Samuel Hahnemann, elevated St. John's wort to a major homeopathic remedy, and it is found in every homeopathic first-aid kit for accidents, injury to the nerves, insect bites, and to promote wound healing. St. John's wort tincture washes and cleans cuts and wounds, inhibits infection, and hastens the healing process, especially in areas rich in nerves. The English physician Dorothy Shepherd said: "I much prefer *hypericum* tincture, applied locally, to any of the modern antiseptics; it does not destroy the healthy tissues and healthy cells; it cleans up dirty septic wounds; it eases inflammation in septic fingers [and] boils. . . . Lacerated crushed fingers and hands remain surgically clean and antiseptic, and heal rapidly."[28] We now know that this esteemed plant has antibacterial and antiviral properties.

Modern herbalists value St. John's wort, using it for coughs, female problems, anxiety, and depression, and they share the homeopaths' enthusiasm for using it externally. One interesting herbal application: St. John's wort eases fatigue, anxiety, and depression, an application recently validated by research. It seems to work with brain chemicals much like prescription antidepressants but without the side effects. In this capacity, St. John's wort has recently become a superstar of herbalism, but this should not blind us to its prudent use based on sound principles. In holistic herbalism several other remedies and methods are also used to stem depression, most notably diet, exercise, other herbs, and vitamins—depending on the characteristics and needs of the individual. In other words, an herbalist would not reflexively give St. John's wort for every case of anxiety or depression.

For those who are skeptical about the value of St. John's wort for depression, several major studies have confirmed its value. One revealed a positive response in 67 percent of patients compared to 28 percent in a placebo group.[29] Not surprisingly, other uses of the plant are being explored: recent studies have shown that hypericin (a compound in the plant)

28. Dorothy Shepherd, *A Physician's Posy* (New Delhi: Jain Publishing, 1983), p. 96.

29. *Journal of Geriatric Psychiatry and Neurology* 7 (1994).

has antiviral activity. Our humble little friend is now being researched for AIDS treatment, attention deficit disorder, obesity, and even cancer.

First Aid. Tincture, ointment, and oil; used to clean and heal cuts, skin, and nerves, and to calm the nervous system. This remedy also can be used on bites, bruises, stings, and burns—a major first-aid remedy.

Primary Uses. Herbalists currently use this herb for coughs, to expel phlegm, for bronchitis, cystitis, nervous exhaustion, PMS, restlessness, mild anxiety, and depression.

Health Promotion. This herb has definite health-promoting qualities.

Doses. Extract and capsules, recommended doses, but for anxiety and depression most agree that it should be taken for at least 3 months to experience its full benefits, and some authorities claim that standardized St. John's wort is preferable, often 300 milligrams 3 times daily. The tea, made from the fresh dried flowers, is a superb remedy for the nervous system. However, St. John's wort is not a cure-all; indiscriminate use of this plant is now common.

Caution. A safe herb within therapeutic guidelines. However, in a few people the remedy might promote allergic skin response when overexposed to sunlight—discontinue use. Those people with serious anxiety or depression should first consult a physician before using this herb, or while taking medications for anxiety or depression.

Complementary Remedies. Other herbs have a reputation for easing mild anxiety, depression, "blues," sadness, and the fatigue that often precedes many cases of sadness and depression. These include lemon balm, the ginsengs, rosemary, damiana, ginkgo, schisandra, rhemmania, he shou wu, and even the humble dandelion. In Oriental medicine there are about five basic causes of depression, each of which requires a different herbal formula, and in Western medicine causes of depression vary and should be diagnosed by a physician.

SAW PALMETTO
Serenoa repens

SOUTHERN HERB BECOMES
INTERNATIONAL MEDICINE

Along with echinacea, goldenseal, and American ginseng, saw palmetto is an American medicine of unusual distinction. This powerful healer, a favorite of Indian tribes in the Deep South, is extracted from the berries of a small palm tree that grows along the coastal region from South Carolina to Florida. Like schisandra berries of China, this herb is a gentle tonic for the whole body, particularly the kidneys and sex organs. Seminoles and other Indians had used this remedy for centuries by the time the first white settlers arrived in Florida and Georgia. African American healers adopted this remedy, and in the nineteenth century saw palmetto was adopted by homeopaths and Eclectics. However, until very recently it has been ignored by conventional medicine. All over our planet, herbalists and homeopaths still commonly use this plant, and recently research has demonstrated its effectiveness, resulting in increased popularity. In fact, saw palmetto has been catapulted from being an obscure Southern herbal folk remedy to being an international herb of some repute.

Saw palmetto is presently used for enlargement of the

prostate gland, called benign prostatic hyperplasia (BPH) in conventional medicine. The prostate gland, a tiny organ located behind the testicles, enlarges in 60 percent of men between forty-nine and fifty-nine years old. This problem can cause painful dribbling and/or frequent urination. The cost for hospital care and surgery for this condition is estimated to be over one billion dollars a year. Surgery, while necessary in some cases, can produce complications and scar tissue. Furthermore, the chronically inflamed prostate gland can become cancerous, a relatively common form of cancer in American males. This condition should not be self-diagnosed, and men who suspect this problem, should not treat themselves. They should seek professional advice.

Saw palmetto shows great promise for the treatment of prostate problems in men. Many double-blind studies, mostly in Europe, have demonstrated the powerful healing benefits of this plant. All of a sudden another great American herb is "validated"; but a hundred years ago the homeopath doctor, William Boericke, wrote that this herb alleviates problems of the prostate gland, particularly inflammation and enlargement, as well as loss of sexual power. The nineteenth-century herbal physicians also used it for similar purposes, and in fact in *The Eclectic Materia Medica*, Dr. Felter mentions it specifically for painful urination and prostatic enlargement. In the reductionist climate of contemporary medicine, saw palmetto has been whittled down to being a drug for the prostate, where traditionally it has been a "terrain" medicine for the urogenital region. Herbalists respect it for its broad healing powers and also use it for women. It has some tonic and adaptogen properties that should not be ignored.

Saw palmetto is a favorite remedy in Europe. Most notably, this healing berry contains an oil with a variety of fatty acids and phytosterols responsible for its healing effects. Standardized extracts might feature these prime compounds, but saw palmetto also contains many other therapeutic constituents, including minerals, vitamins, and important ingredient(s) yet to be identified.

Primary Uses. The German Commission E recommends saw palmetto for prostate complaints and irritable bladder. Herbalists recommend this herb for male and female infertility, to improve sex life, and as general tonic for both men and women. An unsubstantiated herbal use: it has been given to skinny people to "fatten them up" and to women who want to enlarge their breasts; also used for breathing problems, coughs, and asthma, and urinary irritation in both sexes.

Health Promotion. Potential for both men and women.

Doses. Extract and capsules; recommended doses 2 to 3 times a day, taken for several weeks or more. Many herbalists prefer the standardized extracts of this herb. Few problems have been reported with this beneficent herb when taken within reasonable guidelines. The dried berry decoction is a good way to benefit from this healing plant, or tea made from powdered berry.

Caution. A medical doctor must examine men with prostate and urine problems; these include painful urination, passing blood, and excessive, chronic night urination.

Complementary Remedies. The African herb pygeum shows great promise in treating prostate problems. Saw palmetto is found in synergistic formulas with bearberry, bucchu, nettle root, pygeum, and other herbs.

SCHISANDRA
Schisandra chinesis
Wu wei zi

ORIENTAL HERB FOR MEN AND WOMEN

While not well known in the West, schisandra is a famous Oriental medicine in the same class as ginseng and dong quai. Schisandra, a rare ornamental vine in America, is a beautiful sight to admire: the lush green vines are decorated with clusters of miniature red berries. Schisandra berries are found in Chinese herb stores and are increasingly common in health food stores in extracts and formulas. The tart berries, called five-taste fruits in China, are unusual in that they contain the five flavors: sweet, sour, bitter, pungent, and hot, and thus are considered a "balanced" medicine. This beneficial medicine has a long history of use in the Orient, first mentioned in the primary class of herbs in the ancient *Shen Nong Ben Cao Jing.* Li Shi Zhen, one of the great herbal scholars of world history, writes about this premier herb in his 1596 classic, *Ben Cao Gang Mu.*

Health Benefits. Schisandra is a major herb to treat deficient kidney yin, a disharmony pattern that produces nervousness, forgetfulness, and low back pain. It calms the body, nourishes, and acts as an adaptogen. In ancient China, schisandra was valued by the emperors, royal ladies, and, of course, the common people. Traditionally, Chinese women have cherished schisandra because it enhances beauty, promotes vigor, and improves sex. Clinically, this berry is blended with other herbs for dry coughs, weak lungs, asthma, diarrhea, insomnia, and night sweats.

Schisandra is paired with Siberian ginseng for stress relief and sports endurance. This valued herb is also a liver tonic and assists the whole digestive system. It cleans the blood, making the skin healthier and more radiant. It is a gentle tonic for the nervous system, good for agitation, poor sleep, and nervousness. Scientific research in China has verified many health benefits, including the healing of diseased livers. Active constituents include lignans (particularly schisandran), triterpenic acids, triterpene lactones, essential oil, citric acid, and vitamins C and E. Lignans are currently being researched for their ability to inhibit cancer.

The berries can be purchased at Chinese herb stores and through the mail. A heaping tablespoon of the berries can be soaked in a pot of water for several hours. Throw out the water and rinse the berries, add 2 fresh cups of water and a tablespoon of lycii berries. Simmer for 15 minutes. Drink daily for several weeks as a general tonic. It is quite tasty.

Primary Uses. Nervousness, restlessness, fatigue, colds, coughing, to improve mental alertness and poor liver functioning.

Health Promotion. Clearly a good candidate for health promotion and well-being. In China, schisandra is used alone and in formulas for stamina and sexual energy.

Doses. Extract, as directed, synergistic formulas, or teas. A typical dose could be 15 to 20 drops of extract in half a cup of water 2 or 3 times daily for several weeks.

Complementary Remedies. Milk thistle, saw palmetto, motherwort, he shou wu, and ligustrum.

Caution. Avoid during pregnancy, fevers, and rashes.

Note. For scientific data on schisandra, see *Clinical Applications of Ayurvedic and Chinese Herbs*, by Kerry Bone (Warwick, Australia: Phytotherapy Press, 1996).

TEA TREE OIL
Melaleuca alternifolia

AUSTRALIAN POWER HERB

One of the more useful power herbs for home use, tea tree is the essential oil of a tree that grows in damp swamps of New South Wales, Australia. Well adapted to a challenging environment, this tree has developed potent compounds to survive an abundance of parasites, fungus, and bacteria. Utilized by aborigines for thousands of years, tea tree oil is now recognized in Australia for its antiseptic and cleansing qualities. It is an all-purpose cleanser for the skin, mouth, and mucous membranes and is often found in "bush" oils to treat bites and stings. Today this herb, produced commercially in Australian plantations, is exported all over the globe. Tea tree oil is a bona fide healer, a germicide and antiseptic used for a variety of ailments. It has been researched extensively, and double-blind tests have found it effective in fungal infections, acne, and insect bites and even as an antibiotic.

In the past decades tea tree oil has spread far beyond the borders of Australia to join a select pantheon of global power herbs. Some marketing hype has exaggerated its therapeutic benefit. It is not a cure-all, but it is one of the most valuable natural medicines for the skin. Nonetheless, this highly concentrated essential oil should only be used sparingly for external problems, and internal use should be under the advice of a health professional. This pungent, cleansing oil makes an excellent antiseptic for cuts, bites, stings, and fungal problems. Recently, Australian quality standards for tea tree oil have been established. They recommend that a component known as terpinen-4-ol should constitute 30 percent or more of the oil, with less than 15 percent cineole, a compound that compromises the quality of the oil.

First Aid. Cleans and benefits the skin; superb for fungal problems, insect bites and stings, minor cuts and abrasions, acne, and itchy skin. This dynamic oil penetrates deeply into the lower levels of skin where pernicious bacteria can cause infection. Itchy skin, nail infections, skin rashes, and foot odor are other problems that can be helped by this superremedy.

Doses. Tea tree oil is used sparingly as directed; often a couple of drops will suffice, and like other essential oils it can be diluted with water or a bland vegetable oil. Tea tree oil should not be applied full strength on broken skin. It is also available in creams, shampoos, soaps, lotions, and antiseptic solutions.

Oily or irritated skin: use antiseptic solution.

Sprain and joint pain: blend 3 to 6 drops with half a cup of a bland vegetable oil and massage into needy area.

For athlete's foot: clean area with antifungal soap, dry, and apply the pure oil or the cream twice daily.

For fungal problems, warts, insect bites, and boils: dab pure oil with Q-Tip twice daily.

Acne or pimples: clean skin with calendula or tea tree soap. Dab on pure oil to needed spot, or add a few drops of pure oil to warm water, mix well, and rinse the affected area.

Sore gums, cold sores, and sore throats: add 3 to 6 drops to half a cup of water, mix well, rinse out mouth and spit out, and repeat when needed.

Sinus problems or congestion: add 10 drops of pure oil to steam bath or vaporizer.

Lice, fleas, and ticks do not like tea tree oil.

Sunburn: tea tree cream.

Caution. Do not use tea tree oil internally. For those with sensitive skin, test the skin with a drop before applying, cover with a Band-Aid, and see if there is a skin reaction. Use caution with pure oil on red, damaged, or inflamed skin. Pregnant women can use the diluted solution on the skin. Do not use near eyes, as it can cause irritation. A few people might experience an allergic reaction on use; discontinue. See a physician for unusual or persistent skin problems.

Complementary Remedies. Thyme essential oil is also an effective cleanser and antiseptic.

TURMERIC
Curcuma longa

THERAPEUTIC KITCHEN SPICE

It is only fitting to include a major herb from India in this book. The Ayurvedic medical system of India is one of the most durable on this planet, having been in existence for several thousand years, and its compendium of medicinal plants is stupendous. A good number of the herbs in this book are used in Ayurveda, but turmeric until quite recently was not known in the West as a medicine. Today, because of clinical experience and research, turmeric is becoming one of the superstars of global herbal medicine because of its potent healing qualities.

Turmeric, which favors moist hot tropics, is related to ginger. From a knobby tuber emerges a handsome tuft of shiny lanceolate leaves, often 2 to 3 feet tall, and pretty yellow white flowers. The tuberous rhizomes are the source of the medicine. In India and the Far East, vast amounts of turmeric are grown yearly for local use and exportation. Turmeric, slightly bitter and pungent, is a common kitchen spice, particularly in Indian curries, as well as an essential ingredient in Worcestershire sauce. This spice, however, is not hot like cayenne and does not irritate the digestive tract. Turmeric is also an important dye, well known for its bright yellow colors. The yellow color is due to curcumin, also responsible for the color of much commercial mustard. Recently it has been discovered that curcumin is an antioxidant, perhaps even more potent than vitamins C and E.

Health Benefits. In the West one of the first reports of turmeric was from the explorer Marco Polo. In China he observed a yellow plant powder that resembled saffron, one of the most expensive, pound for pound, spices in the world. Because it is much cheaper, turmeric was considered a poor man's saffron. The poor men were luckier than they realized. Turmeric, used in Ayurvedic and Chinese medicine for hundreds of years, is still considered a valuable remedy in these traditions. It properties are cooling, cleansing, and detoxifying, with affinities for the blood, liver, and whole digestive system, and it has been used by Oriental herbalists for a variety of chronic diseases, including cancer. There is no evidence that turmeric can cure cancer, but it has been commonly employed as an adjunct treatment. Cancer treatment in Oriental medicine, directed toward the person and the disease, includes a broad spectrum of modalities, including conventional medicine, nutrition, and herbal formulas.

Like milk thistle and schisandra, turmeric increases production of liver enzymes that metabolize dangerous toxins. Contemporary studies have revealed that the traditional respect for this therapeutic spice is well founded. Turmeric can inhibit the development of cancer, and, as several studies suggest, it has the potential to promote cancer regression. In its anti-inflammatory effects, turmeric is quite formidable. Furthermore, studies have supported traditional uses for this medicine in digestive and liver conditions. The German Commission E reports a good handful of medicinal actions, including antitumor, antiseptic, and anti-inflammatory. This power herb is loaded with therapeutic properties.

First Aid. Turmeric is a valuable external poultice or ointment for sprains, strains, and local inflammations. It can also be taken internally for these conditions.

Primary Uses. In herbal medicine turmeric is utilized alone and in formulas for a wide variety of diseases, including atherosclerosis, fevers, hepatitis, jaundice, gallstones, ulcers, irritable stomach and intestines, cysts, fibroids, tumors, swellings, inflammations, arthritis, chronic fevers, painful menstrual cramps, abdominal masses, and bruises. Of course, for any medical condition professional guidance should be sought.

Health Promotion. Clearly turmeric, the kitchen spice, should be consumed liberally in daily diet. It does not overwhelm dishes like cayenne. At least a quarter of a teaspoon can be added to soups, stews, and vegetable dishes, or follow the recipe.

Doses. Besides the kitchen uses, turmeric can be taken as capsules, extracts, and synergistic formulas. Typical dose: 1 capsule, 300 to 400 milligrams, up to 3 times a day. For the deep liver cleansing and for arthritis, several excellent synergistic formulas are now available.

Cautions. A safe natural medicine, but those with gallstones should seek professional advice before using medicinal portions of turmeric.

Complementary Remedies. Barberry, milk thistle,

schisandra, artichoke leaf, celandine, baikal skullcap (Chinese remedy), and dandelion root.

VALERIAN
Valeriana officinalis

HERBAL TRANQUILIZER

Valerian is an ancient medicinal plant very much alive in the modern world. The history of valerian is particularly rich because it was known to Egyptians, Greeks, and Romans, and during the Middle Ages it was a popular medicine, even acquiring the name *heal all*. Some writers say that the origin of its name is the Latin word *valere*, which means to be in health. Medieval apothecaries used valerian for headaches, insomnia, hysteria, epilepsy, cramping, and other nervous conditions. American Indians valued valerian, as did the nineteenth-century American herbal doctors, the Eclectics; one of their luminaries, Dr. Felter, says of the plant, "It is one of the best of calmatives for that collective condition termed nervousness."[30] As usual, time has proven Dr. Felter right.

The root, the source of the medicine, produces a tall, stately plant that flourishes in the garden. Each June the stalks, 5 or 6 feet tall, produce beautiful umbrellas of tiny white (tinged with pink) flowers that have a somewhat intoxicating aroma said to attract cats and other animals. Recently it has been determined that valerian contains compounds similar to catnip. In fact one version of the story of the Pied Piper of Hamelin has him attracting the rats and the children of the town with music and the hypnotic aroma of valerian

30. Felter, *The Eclectic Materia Medica*.

roots. This handsome herb, a perennial available at many garden stores, is an easy one to add to the garden. Once it has found a good spot it hunkers down and spreads each year and is virtually indestructible.

Health Benefits. Probably the major relaxant of herbalism, this global power herb is used for mild anxiety, nervousness, and sleep problems. Science has effectively dispelled any lingering fancies that this plant is a hoax; valerian is a safe and effective medicine. Two important compounds found in valerian, valepotriates and valeric acid, are unique to the plant. Valerian extracts seem to work by enhancing the activity of the gammaminobutyric acid (GABA), a major inhibitory neurotransmitter. Valerian acts as a tranquilizer on the nervous system in times of agitation and curiously enough as a stimulant in cases of extreme fatigue. Unlike chemical sedatives (for instance, valium) and other benzodiazepine drugs, valerian does not impair mental functioning, cause hangovers, or create a physical addiction. Furthermore, it does not interfere with the stages of sleep like prescription drugs.

First Aid. It can be used for agitation and sleeplessness following any emotional or physical trauma.

Primary Uses. This effective plant medicine is approved by the German Commission E for restlessness and sleep disorders caused by nervous conditions. It has some use in mild cases of anxiety and is also found in formulas for cramping, anxiety, and pain.

Doses. Adult: 20 to 30 drops of extract in water before retiring, which can be repeated once if awakened, or 1 to 2 capsules or tablets, as directed; repeated large doses are definitely not better. For those who are chronically exhausted, other herbs to support the nervous system are preferable initially. Synergistic formulas (valerian works well with kava kava) are sometimes the best way to utilize this medicine. This is *not* an herb for the long term; use only when needed.

Cautions. Valerian is a safe, nonaddictive medicine. However, a small minority do not respond well; it makes them more restless. As an alternative, other herbal remedies can be tried. Valerian does not interfere with driving or operating heavy machinery and can be used by pregnant women. Do *not* take valerian with alcohol, antidepressants, or sleep-inducing drugs and, as with any medicine, do not exceed the recommended doses.

Complementary Remedies. Passionflower, despite its name, is milder and sometimes preferable to valerian. For children lemon balm and passionflower are good herbs for relaxation. Reishi, a power herb, is another remedy for sleep problems, as is hops and St. John's wort.

VITEX
Vitex agnus-castus

WOMAN'S REMEDY

Vitex, or chaste tree, is a recently revived power herb in Europe. This extraordinary healing plant has a curious and intricate history. Native to the Mediterranean region, vitex is a small deciduous tree, a kind of wild lilac that bears fragrant pink-violet flowers and arrays of light green, pointed leaves. The medicine is produced from berries (and leaves) that are small and hard, similar to a peppercorn. Vitex has also been called chasteberry, chaste tree, and monk's pepper. The curious name *monk's pepper* came about because at monasteries the dried hard fruit was ground and sprinkled on the meals like a pepper. Apparently, it was used to decrease the libido of the monks. Whether this property is a fact remains a question; not in question is that vitex is a major remedy for women.

Well known in the Mediterranean world, vitex has been used by herbalists and physicians since ancient times, mostly for balancing the menstrual cycle of women. Hippocrates, Pliny, and countless others have respected this natural medicine, but it has not been known in America until quite recently.

Health Benefits. Vitex contains an array of potentially healing compounds, including one that has a progesterone-like effect. Traditionally herbalists have also used this herb to promote fertility and reduce fibroids, uses that have not yet been verified by modern science. In modern clinics, the use of vitex centers around the menstrual cycle. PMS, menopause, and irregular periods can be relieved by vitex. This remarkable plant medicine also reduces the anxieties, irritability, and nervousness often associated with menstrual cycles. This is a safe herb with no known toxicity, an all-purpose herb for women. Clinically prescribed vitex is a viable, safe, and natural alternative to hormone replacement therapy. Herbalists often combine it with other herbs and food supplements like evening primrose oil. The German Commission E recognizes vitex; it is a common herb in European clinics. In one European clinical study a vitex tincture was tested on 1,571 women with menstrual disorders and PMS and was found to eliminate or alleviate symptoms in 90 percent of the women.

Primary Uses. Hot flashes, night sweats, swelling of the breasts, anxiety, PMS, irregular periods, amenorrhea, and menopause. European herbalists also use this herb (often in synergistic formulas) to promote fertility and decrease fibroids.

Health Promotion. This herb has marked health-promotion effects for women.

Doses. Extracts, tablets, and capsules, as recommended; for example, 40 drops of extract, once daily, for 3 to 18 months. To achieve the best benefit for menstrual irregularities, it should be taken for at least 3 months. Please consult an herbalist for specific doses when using the herb for the long term.

Complementary Remedies. Dong quai, motherwort, raspberry, black cohosh, flaxseed, and primrose oil.

Caution. Contraindicated in pregnancy or lactation. Very occasionally itching and rashes can result from vitex therapy—discontinue use or consult a health professional.

Note. See D. Brown, *"Vitex agnus-castus,"* clinical monograph, *Quarterly Review of Natural Medicines* (Summer 1994): 111–21.

PART FOUR

HERBAL EXTRAS

A brief review follows of major herbs not discussed in this book and up-and-coming herbs that few people have heard about. Some of these valuable plant medicines need serious consideration for more research and clinical use.

Black haw (*Viburnum prunifolium*). An important female herb for menstrual problems and pains.

Black walnut (*Juglans nigra*). An old herbal standby, healing for the digestive tract, with antifungal properties.

Cat's claw (*Uncaria tomentosa*). A rain forest herb with a growing reputation for immune enhancement and disease prevention, used for cancer, arthritis, and AIDS.

Chaparral (*Larrea* spp.). Important detoxifying herb that has a history of use for chronic diseases and cancer—its use is restricted to health professionals.

Damiana (*Turnera aphrodisiaca*). Power herb from Central America; damiana supports the nervous system and the sexual functions.

Fenugreek (*Trigonella foenumgraecum*). An ancient herbal medicine and spice now finding use for high cholesterol, diabetes, and other diseases of civilization.

Motherwort (*Leonurus cardiaca*). A traditional herb for women that has some important applications in the modern world.

Osha (*Ligusticum porteri*). Rocky Mountain herb with antiviral properties, often used for coughs and sore throats.

Thyme (*Thymus vulgaris*). A therapeutic garden herb for coughs, colds, digestive problems, and gentle immune stimulus.

Yarrow (*Achillea millefolium*). Another garden herb, excellent for digestion, colds, and other common problems.

Yerba Santa (*Eriodictyon californica*). Important herb for the lungs, sinuses, and coughs.

Yucca (*Yucca liliaceaea*). A remedy of the southwest Indians; shows promise in arthritic conditions.

PART FIVE

POWER HERBS FOR DISEASE PREVENTION AND HEALTH PROMOTION

This part offers remedies and suggestions for common everyday health problems and health promotion. These suggestions are not meant to replace the good and necessary care of doctors and are not intended for serious and chronic diseases. For medical advice on herbal medicines, seek a professional herbalist.

Many symptoms should send us to the proper health care. These include high fever, any prolonged or severe bleeding, unusual changes in stools, any unusual lumps or bumps, difficulty breathing, severe headaches, head or eye injury, relentless vomiting and cramping, and sharp recurring pains.

For instructions about using herbal remedies, review part 2. Most of the herbs referenced in this section are power herbs. The most appropriate remedy can be studied for possible use.

ACCIDENTS AND TRAUMA. For minor accidents or postmedical treatment after major accidents, the following remedies can be helpful: arnica, valerian, St. John's wort, kava kava, chamomile, ligustrum, ginseng, or calendula.

AGING. see *Longevity*.

ALLERGIES. Allergies, a complex problem, require advice from an herbalist, but a handful of the power herbs can alleviate symptoms: milk thistle, dandelion, *eyebright*, *nettle*, goldenseal, *elderberry tea*, and feverfew.

ANXIETY AND NERVOUSNESS. For simple everyday anxiety and nervousness that does not require medical attention: valerian, reishi, schisandra, kava kava, skullcap, chamomile, damiana, passionflower, or St. John's wort. Herbal tea combinations are highly recommended for the home. Anyone who feels the need to use any of these herbs for the long term should see a health professional for advice.

ARTHRITIS. Joint pain. Anyone suffering from painful joints should be cognizant of the fact that there are multiple solutions, including an initial medical checkup, diet, exercise, and gentle stretching. Helpful herbal remedies include: *black cohosh*, arnica, boneset, feverfew, *turmeric*, devil's claw, yucca, barberry, flaxseed oil, and fresh greens. Commercial formulas of these and other herbs can be tried for up to two or three weeks, or as suggested on labels. For stubborn cases of arthritis, I suggest dietary changes along with professional herbal advice, as well as massage and acupuncture.

BACKACHE. Simple everyday backaches due to muscular stress and strain: heat or ice—ice for inflammation. *Arnica* ointment can be helpful for stiffness and muscular soreness due to overexertion. Capsicum (red pepper)–based ointments provide heat and some relief from backache that is better with heat and worse in damp weather. Very important: sensible lifting, a stretching routine, baths and massage, and in difficult cases, a medical checkup. See the herbs under *Sports injury*.

BITES AND STINGS. Tea tree oil or garlic juice; internal: echinacea, eyebright, or nettle leaf formulas. Baking soda: moistened and applied to bites—a good old home remedy. For a few very sensitive people, insect bites can be a medical emergency. Symptoms to watch out for: difficult breathing, confusion, convulsions, loss of consciousness, rapid red swelling, or constriction in throat.

BLADDER INFECTION. See *Urinary tract infection*.

BRUISES. External: arnica, St. John's wort, or tea tree oil; internal: ginkgo, gotu kola, or bilberry.

BURNS. For simple, small burns that do not require medical attention: *Aloe* or *calendula*. Do *not* apply butter or thick ointments in the initial period of a burn. Do not use ice on burned skin. Homeopathic *nettle*—*Urtica urens*—makes an excellent lotion or tincture for burns that itch and sting. Second- and third-degree burns, where skin is broken, blistered, and shiny, need immediate medical attention.

CANCER. Anyone with cancer must see a health professional if he or she wants to benefit from medicinal herbs. As an adjunct to comprehensive treatment, remedies include: maitake, reishi, ginseng, licorice, ligustrum, goldenseal, chaparral, milk thistle, burdock, greens, red clover, barberry, St. John's wort, he shou wu, schisandra, turmeric, and green tea. Specialized synergistic formulas are available, depending on the needs of the patient. There are no magic herbs to cure cancer, but herbal medicines can assist in the healing of cancer patients.

CANKER SORES. Rinse mouth with tincture of myrrh, bilberry, or diluted tea tree oil. Healthy foods include onions, garlic, greens like broccoli, and yogurt. Avoid citrus, coffee (any stimulants), sugar, and junk food in general. Apply myrrh locally with a Q-Tip.

CHILDREN'S HERBS. These include echinacea, arnica, calendula, elderberry, astragalus, elecampane, peppermint, lemon balm, and chamomile. Infants require medical advice. Excellent synergistic formulas are available for children; follow the recommendations of an herbalist or the product guide. Children respond very well to herbal remedies and to aromatic massage oils.

COMMON COLD. Echinacea, elderberry, ginger, goldenseal, schisandra, chamomile, hyssop, thyme, or boneset. Colds, especially the damp and chilly ones with fluent clear discharge, respond well to frequent warm herbal teas—ginger tea is a good one. Garlic, echinacea, and ginger are cold preventatives. A wonderful tea combination is elderflower, peppermint, and yarrow.

CONSTIPATION. Recommended are the following. (1) A fiber diet with plenty of fruits, whole grains, and vegetables. (2) Herbs include *senna*, which have chemicals in them that really do stimulate the bowels, so they should not be used habitually. Use these cautiously or as directed by a health professional. *Psyllium* is a seed that expands when moist and increases bowel motility and should be used as directed with plenty of water. (3) *Exercise.* (4) Some medical drugs, antihistamines, diuretics, and antidepressants can cause constipation—consult a drug reference book or pharmacist. *Caution.* Any person with chronic bowel problems should consult a physician before taking any herbal medicines. Any chronic constipation or changes of color in bowels or bleeding can be a warning to see a physician.

COUGH. Most coughing is a common reflex action of the body, often the result of cold, flu, or allergy, but some persistent or violent coughs are warning signs that should be heeded. Herbal teas and syrups can soothe simple coughs. Common herbs: elderberry, elecampane, licorice, thyme, schisandra, hyssop, yarrow, and yerba santa. Essential oils, blended with a bland vegetable oil, can be rubbed on the chest and back: eucalyptus, tea tree, and myrrh are some of the best, especially when combined with acupressure and massage on the upper back and shoulders.

Rudolf Weiss (*Herbal Medicine*) gives the following herbal tea for acute, dry coughs: mullein, coltsfoot, marsh mallow, and anise seed, equal parts totaling 2 teaspoons, in a cup of boiling water. Cover and infuse for 20 minutes and drink several times a day, with honey if desired. For dry, weak, persistent coughs: American ginseng. For thick mucous coughs: elecampane formulas; other good formulas contain thyme, horehound, or mullein.

See your doctor if the cough lasts for more than 7 days, or if there is rusty, green, or yellow phlegm, high fever, shortness of breath, body aches, weight loss, chest pains, or severe headache. Coughing blood requires a medical exam.

CRAMPS. Muscle cramping: dong quai formulas, ginkgo, and dandelion formulas. Cramps can be a sign of deficiency of calcium or potassium in the diet: try eating more vegetable greens, brown rice, oatmeal, sesame seeds, and fruits like banana, and less salt, fried foods, and saturated fats. External: arnica, chamomile, or St. John's wort.

CUTS AND ABRASIONS. Clean thoroughly with soap and

warm water, and apply topically: calendula or St. John's wort tincture. Chamomile is another valued remedy. Lotions and ointments of these herbs are highly recommended to soothe and heal the skin. In serious cases of cuts or infections with heavy bleeding, swelling, pain, redness, and pus, always consult a doctor. Hydrogen peroxide is also a good cleanser and disinfectant.

DIARRHEA. Emotional distress, reactions to food, and medications are some of the causes of diarrhea. Herbs that can help simple cases of this condition include psyllium, red raspberry, bilberry, ginger, or chamomile. Drink plenty of liquids. Slippery elm is a soothing herb for the intestines. Foods include raw green apples, bananas, papaya, applesauce, oats, and yogurt. Milk products can be allergenic, as can wheat products. Ingest yogurt or acidophilus for diarrhea brought on by antibiotics or reactions to food. *Cautions.* Diarrhea that lasts for more than a few days needs a medical exam, as does bloody, painful, or violent diarrhea. Recurrent diarrhea can be a sign of irritable bowel syndrome (alternating with constipation), colitis, or gastroenteritis (diarrhea alternating with vomiting)—see a physician.

DRUG DETOX. Along with counseling and medical guidance, the following herbs are known to be useful: St. John's wort, milk thistle, oat extract, ligustrum, licorice, schisandra, reishi, chamomile, or gotu kola. Consult an herbalist for instructions.

EARACHE. For simple earaches unaccompanied by high fever and pain, the following remedies have proven helpful. A medical exam is important with the ears. (1) A drop or two of *mullein oil* in ear. If not available, try garlic juice (mixed with a little olive oil). Put 1 to 3 drops in ear every 4 hours for a day or two, but never if the eardrum is punctured. White vinegar is a home remedy for washing out the ear. After swimming or any potential exposure, take the dropperful of vinegar, squeeze into ear, tilt head so solution reaches the bottom of the ear, and then let the liquid drain out. (2) Herbs include goldenseal, pau d'arco, and echinacea. Use caution with any pain or discharge from ears, or dizziness or ringing in ears— see a doctor.

EYES. Specific herbs for eyestrain (for computer operators and bookworms): bilberry, eyebright, schisandra, and milk thistle.

FATIGUE AND EXHAUSTION. Any unusual, recurrent, or long-term case of fatigue should be examined by a doctor. Chronic fatigue or exhaustion unrelated to overwork, restless sleep, or excess exercise can be a warning sign that should be heeded. Chronic tiredness is often related to poor organ functioning, such as an overburdened liver or intestine. An herbalist might diagnose a congested liver and prescribe 2 or 3 weeks of special diet and liver cleansing herbs.

These suggestions for fatigue or exhaustion relate to athletes who overdo it or anyone burdened by a period of too much work or distress. Common sense about a healthy diet and not too many stimulants is important: excess coffee, rich food, and lack of sleep can lead to fatigue. Of course, excess emotional and mental stress can be a major contribution. Chief remedies for deficient energy: the ginsengs, gotu kola, licorice, and astragalus; dandelion root is a gentle tonic; St. John's wort tea, particularly for those who are nervous and anxious. Other herbs to consider include damiana, he shou wu, schisandra, ligustrum, and ginkgo.

FEMALE REMEDIES. Vitex, schisandra, he shou wu,

raspberry, black and blue cohosh, primrose oil, olive oil, milk thistle, thyme, greens, cramp bark, chamomile, soybean products, and dong quai—among the best of many. Herbal remedies can help women in many ways: beauty, energy, healthy skin, hormone cycles, sexual health, and overall well-being.

FEVER. The suggestions provided here are for short-term, low fevers. Herbs: echinacea, boneset, elderflower, peppermint, and chamomile. If a tea is made from one or a formula of these herbs, prepare a strong potion and ingest a modest amount several times through the course of the day. Drink plenty of fluid, rest, and reduce solid, greasy, and spicy foods. Most often, it is best to let a moderate fever run its course without too much tampering with drugs, but fevers, especially with children, must be watched carefully. A cool compress on the forehead as well as a tepid upper body wash can help cool the body. Make sure you keep a thermometer in your medicine cabinet, because fevers over 103 degrees need monitoring and possible medical attention.

FLU. Boneset, echinacea, or *elderberry*: strong, repeated teas.

FUNGAL INFECTIONS. External: tea tree oil, black walnut, or goldenseal (powder, ointment, or extract); internal: garlic, basil tea, elecampane, *black walnut, pau d'arco,* turmeric, myrrh, or olive leaf extract.

GAS. Can be corrected by eating more slowly and consuming a sensible, balanced diet. Eating on the run or while emotionally upset will help instigate digestive wind! Do not avoid fiber-rich foods, vegetables, and fruit. Herbs that calm the stomach and intestines include fennel, coriander, and caraway—all common kitchen herbs. Seeds can be chewed, or use teas. Chamomile and peppermint, two power herbs, are good for many problems of the digestive system. Charcoal tablets, available at the health food store, are a universal standby. Kitchen remedy: burnt toast. Seek medical attention for chronic gas or gas accompanied by any pains, weight loss, fever, and swelling. Food allergies, laxatives, antacids, antibiotics, and other drugs can disrupt the digestive system.

GUMS AND MOUTH. Tea tree oil mouthwash, echinacea, pau d'arco, bilberry, myrrh, chamomile, or goldenseal. Herbal mouthwashes of these herbs can be purchased.

HAY FEVER. A problem that often requires professional advice from an herbalist, naturopath, or homeopath. Remedies that can help relieve symptoms: eyebright (often with synergistic herbs), nettle leaf, or elderflower formulas; dandelion, red root/lymph combinations can also be helpful. A rich diet of saturated fats, milk products, and sugar seems to aggravate allergies like hay fever, and, in fact, herbalists often advise nutritional changes along with herbal therapy.

HEADACHE. Any stubborn, long-term, or painful headaches require medical examination, but for simple everyday stress headaches the following remedies can offer positive relief: *feverfew, peppermint, skullcap,* chamomile, or milk thistle. If using a tea make a strong 4 cups' worth and drink 1 cup 2 or 3 times daily. Herbal baths are helpful, as well as massages of the head, neck, and shoulders. A few drops of peppermint oil can be rubbed into the side or back of the scalp.

HEART AND CARDIOVASCULAR. Anyone with suspected or diagnosed heart or blood pressure problems should consult a physician before using medicinal potions of herbs. There are several good herbs for the heart and the blood vessels, including hawthorn, garlic, he shou wu, ginseng, olive oil, greens, green tea, reishi, soy foods, and guggul (see myrrh). Most important, those concerned should seriously examine their diet (see olive oil and greens), exercise, and consult a professional.

HEMORRHOIDS. The main sources of this problem are a rich diet, lack of fiber, straining while evacuating, lack of exercise, and sedentary lifestyle. Constipation or diarrhea most often precedes hemorrhoids. Pregnant women are also susceptible to hemorrhoids. Seek constitutional care. Local remedies for the hemorrhoids: witch hazel; horse chestnut can be taken internally and externally, as well as fiber supplements (psyllium) and aloe vera juice, vitamin C with flavonoids, and vitamin E.

HIGH CHOLESTEROL. Along with dietary changes and medical checkup, the following herbs may be prescribed by an herbalist: garlic, guggul (see myrrh), he shou wu, psyllium, green tea, reishi or shiitake, or fenugreek.

IMMUNE SYSTEM. The immune system is a complex of factors that protect us from disease factors like pernicious bacteria, viruses, and parasites. Abuses to the immune system are very common in the modern world: recreational drugs, overuse of medical drugs, pollution, excess emotional distress, electromagnetic pollution, inadequate nutrition, and a diet rich in salt, saturated fats, and junk food. There are many strategies to strengthen the immune system. The most important are healthy nutrition, fresh air, exercise, and natural remedies. The immune system is intimately connected to the emotions and thoughts and can be greatly helped when our emotional/mental state is more harmonious and positive. Chronic worry, anger, overthinking, and anxiety can weaken the immune system, particularly when combined with an inadequate diet. Herbal medicines: astragalus, elderberry, American ginseng, garlic, reishi, echinacea, schisandra, ligustrum, pau d'arco, red clover, greens, and many others. Anyone with an immune-related disease should consult a professional before using herbal remedies.

INDIGESTION. A generic term for quite a few very common stomach/intestinal problems. In fact, indigestion is one of the most common disorders that afflict human beings. Symptoms can vary: gas, abdominal pains, heartburn, bloating, belching, vomiting, and mild nausea. Indigestion is most often diet related: eating too fast and/or while under emotional stress or overindulging in rich food. Herbal remedies for the digestion are many. *Chamomile* or *peppermint* (more for bloating and gas) tea can be taken three times daily. A dependable all-around tea is peppermint/ginger. Bitter herbal tonics are often used to improve digestion and decrease heartburn—often containing *gentian* or *ginger.* Fennel, licorice, and fenugreek are other common herbal remedies for a stressed stomach. For chronic indigestion—after a medical checkup—seek stress relief through meditation, herbs, and exercise. A good herbal tea for the stomach and digestive tract: lemon balm, orange peel, chamomile, and peppermint.

Caution. Any severe cramping, vomiting, and pain could be a sign of medical emergency, as could digestive symptoms accompanied by fever, diarrhea, vomiting, bleeding, and any alterations of the color of stools.

INSOMNIA. See *Sleeplesness.*

LONGEVITY. Good wholesome nutrition, exercise, and a happy, creative heart and mind are quite obviously the foundation of longevity. It has been found that most people who live long lives keep active and creative till their last days.

Many of the adaptogenic and liver herbs are considered longevity herbs—in other words, herbs that benefit the body/mind and that could prolong life (as long as there is a healthy, balanced lifestyle and diet). Some premier longevity herbs: ginseng, reishi, schisandra, rehmannia, ligustrum, maitake mushroom, milk thistle, he shou wu, garlic, ginkgo, greens, rosemary, astragalus, suma (South American herb), saw palmetto, green tea, hawthorn, and, in fact, many of the power herbs.

Some of our common foods like greens, carrots, rice, beans, winter squash, soy products, turnips, and onions contain antioxidants that can slow the aging process (see greens and power foods). Recently it was discovered that the folic acid in greens and beans can slow the onset of Alzheimer's disease. Acidophilus, found in fermented foods like yogurt, is essential for good health and long life. Fish, olive, primrose, and other good-quality oils are necessary nutritional supplements to ensure good health (see *Olive oil*). Exercise that tones the joints, muscles, and heart is essential for a long life, as is continued flexibility of the spine through stretching, exercise, acupressure, and massage. The motility and health of the intestines, the quality of the blood, and the vigor of the immune system are of utmost importance in promoting good health and long life. Processed foods, saturated fats, unnecessary chemical drugs, nicotine, excess caffeine, unhealthy sex life (sex should be enjoyable), lack of sleep, overwork, extreme and negative emotions, and lack of exercise can undermine the health of the liver, blood, and body.

MALE REMEDIES. These include saw palmetto, ginseng (all of them), ginkgo, milk thistle, garlic, he shou wu, rehmannia, damiana, greens, and power foods. Sound nutrition, exercise, and herbal medicines are a safe, effective program for men seeking more energy and better health. Herbs like yohimbe or medical drugs that arouse the sex drive should be used cautiously because of possible long-term side effects. For herbs and sexual health, see an herbalist.

MENOPAUSE. It is best to consult a health professional if seeking an alternative to conventional medicine. Effective remedies to consider: vitex, dong quai, vitamin E, motherwort, essential fatty acids, schisandra, red clover, and black cohosh formulas. Nutrition is fundamental to correct the more unpleasant symptoms: a diet high in vegetables, fish, fruit, soybean products and fiber foods, also a limit on coffee and other stimulants, saturated fats, sugar, and junk foods. Yoga, tai chi, acupuncture, and meditation are good adjunct tools. The natural passage of menopause can be greatly eased with good nutrition and herbal remedies.

MENSTRUATION. Many excellent herbs exist for the health of women and for the free passage of the menses. For prolonged painful and irregular menstrual cycle it is best to consult a professional. Some herbs for deficient menstrual cycle (amenorrhea) include *dong quai*, vitex, dandelion, schisandra, myrrh, or red clover formulas to nourish the blood. A vigorous and balanced diet is very important in deficient menstrual cycle. See *PMS*.

MIND. For memory and concentration: ginkgo, gotu kola, ginseng, ligustrum, schisandra, rosemary, St. John's wort, he shou wu, red clover formulas, reishi, or rehmannia. Synergistic formulas are recommended, as well as adequate minerals, B vitamins, and antioxidants. Essential fatty acids are important for the health of the brain and nervous system but will not do much good if the diet is rich in saturated fats, sugars, alcohol, salt, and junk foods. Naturally, exercise of the brain and body are fundamental. Rosemary baths, valued for their gentle invigoration, can be enjoyed regularly.

MOTION SICKNESS. Ginger tea or extract, the old stand-by, works well at sea or in the car. Chamomile or peppermint tea can be helpful; use a strong tea.

MOUTH ULCERS. See *Canker sores.*

MUSCLE PAIN. See *Sports injury.*

PARASITES. This problem requires medical testing to diagnose, but symptoms include lethargy, gas, bloating, and changes in the consistency of the stools and are most common after travel in foreign countries. Some common herbal remedies that can help the body rid itself of parasites include: garlic, goldenseal, pumpkin seed, and black walnut extract; but a professional should be consulted for dosages and specifics.

PMS. Premenstrual syndrome: common symptoms include bloating, swollen tender breasts, fatigue, irritability, and changeable moods. Many good herbs and vitamins can assist in alleviating this unpleasant condition. For recurrent or intense PMS it is best to see a practitioner for a complete program. Herbs: *dong quai*, St. John's wort, *vitex*, false unicorn, and black cohosh; dandelion leaf tea 2 to 3 times a day for fluid retention. Prime nutrients: B-6, B-complex, vitamin E, calcium/magnesium, evening primrose oil (one capsule, 500 milligrams, once daily); helpful are synergistic formulas with these vitamins and herbs. In addition, reduce red meat, sugar, chocolate, and coffee and other stimulants, as well as greasy or cold foods (such as ice cream), and eat plenty of vitamin-rich foods. Saturated fats can be a culprit in PMS. Emotions can be a critical underlying factor, especially suppressed anger or anxiety. Try acupuncture, yoga, therapy, and just plain playfulness.

PROSTATE. Regular checkups are important for men over fifty, especially for those with a family history of cancer or with genitourinary problems. Fifty percent of men over fifty experience some degree of prostatic enlargement. Natural remedies can help incipient prostrate problems, the most common of which is prostatic enlargement, or benign prostatic hyperplasia (BPH). The first signs of this problem include increasing night urination, difficulty in urinating, or dribbling of urine. Any urinary or prostate problems need to be monitored by a doctor, and BPH should not be self-diagnosed. Therapy for prevention: sensible whole foods diet, reduction of poor-quality fats, meat, and alcohol. Common medicinal herbs include: saw palmetto, pygeum, pumpkin seed, nettle root, Chinese ginseng, and pipsissewa. It is best to include essential fatty acids, vitamins C and E, and zinc in this preventative program. Rich sources of zinc include oysters, wheat bran, whole oatmeal, pumpkin and sunflower seeds. Drink plenty of good-quality water. *Caution.* See a physician for urinary retention, or blood in urine.

POISON IVY. The prime symptoms are red itchy skin followed by small blisters that fill with clear liquid. The best cure is prevention. Learn to identify the plants. When contact occurs, immediately wash area with strong soap and water and then wipe with rubbing alcohol—useless if this is done too late. Poison ivy is spread by the irritating oils of the plant. Wash all infected clothing in hot water. Relief from itching: the juice of common plantain (*Plantago major*) or jewelweed. Clay pastes (to which can be added a little goldenseal powder) can be used to draw out toxins, or the old kitchen standby, baking soda paste applied to the affected area. Herbs: goldenseal (external), blood cleansing formula, such as myrrh or dandelion root formulas. Rhus tox, homeopathic poison ivy, is used for reducing incidence of rash; take as prophylactic, 30c twice daily for a few days. Consult a physician for serious cases of poison ivy.

SINUSITIS. An inflammation and pain in sinus cavities above the eyes and around the nose, often with postnasal drip or mucus discharge, difficulty breathing through the nose, as well as local tenderness, pain, and congestion. The common cold or flu and viral or bacterial infections are often involved in sinus problems and often need medical attention. There are remedies that can help in short-term or mild cases. Goldenseal, particularly when there is a yellow, thick nasal discharge; echinacea, eyebright, or elderflower formulas, pau d'arco, astragalus, and ginger. A healing tea includes equal parts echinacea, goldenseal, and marshmallow leaf—drink a cup every two to three hours. Internally: garlic and vitamin C.

An effective home remedy to clear the nasal cavity: inhaling the aromas of herbs like eucalyptus, tea tree oil, or thyme and rubbing aromatic massage oils around the nose acupressure points. For those who suffer from sinus problems and have not tried a steam inhalation treatment, well, your time has come. Place thyme, or eucalyptus tea (or 5 to 10 drops of tea tree oil) into a bowl of hot water and breathe the fumes with a towel draped over the head to capture the steam. *Caution.* If there is a serious fever, severe pain, foul-smelling discharge, or problem in the vicinity of the eyes—seek medical attention.

SLEEPLESSNESS, INSOMNIA, AND RESTLESSNESS. For simple cases of occasional restless nights, the following sug-

gestions can be very helpful. Some simple solutions: do not
drink stimulants, like caffeine drinks, 3 to 4 hours before
going to bed. Engage in vigorous exercise during the day,
not just for 10 minutes but up to an hour. Learn some relaxation exercises with tapes, classes, or books, and do not eat a
large meal within four hours of bedtime. Rising late is not
recommended, or naps. Herbal remedies include valerian,
California poppy, skullcap, hops, reishi, passionflower, or St.
John's wort. Valerian and kava kava formulas are very good.
A soothing passionflower and hops tea (a strong $1/2$ cup) can
be taken one hour before retiring, with the rest of the cup
next to the bed to be used if needed.

SKIN. For dry skin, abrasions, mild burns, and minor
rashes, the following remedies are suggested: calendula, aloe
vera, St. John's wort tincture or oil, olive oil, tea tree cream,
or echinacea. Calendula lotion, cream, or ointment is a good
all-around remedy for skin health.

SORE THROAT. For mild, short-term sore throats: echinacea, elderberry, bilberry, echinacea gargle, thyme, echi-
nacea/goldenseal, and pau d'arco. Tea tree lozenges. Vitamin
C lozenges with zinc and echinacea are a superb combination.

SPORTS INJURY/MUSCLE STRAIN. After a medical
exam, external application: arnica, St. John's wort, turmeric,
or comfrey; internal: turmeric, black cohosh, yucca, ginger, or
Siberian ginseng; formulas with turmeric are highly recommended for muscle and joint inflammation.

STRESS. Generalized stress from overwork or too much
exertion: ginseng (all kinds), reishi, antioxidant vitamin formula with herbs and B vitamins, chamomile, schisandra, he
shou wu, St. John's wort, rehmannia, ligustrum, gotu kola,

kava kava, or valerian. Baths with essential oil of rosemary or lavender are very relaxing. See *Fatigue.*

STOMACH. See *Indigestion.*

SUNBURN. Aloe vera juice, calendula, or St. John's wort lotion or spray. For severe sunburn, see a medical doctor.

TRAVEL SICKNESS. See *Motion sickness.*

ULCERS. Peptic ulcers are internal sores (lesions) that occur as a result of multiple stresses. The lining of the stomach is damaged when the stomach is unable to release protective mucus secretion. To prevent ulcers, licorice, cabbage juice, goldenseal, and peppermint or chamomile tea; but for active ulcers, see a professional herbalist.

URINARY TRACT INFECTION. Often involves harmful bacteria—see a health professional. Helpful preventative herbs include cranberry, unsweetened juice or extracts, barberry, bearberry, goldenseal, or juniper. Synergistic bladder formulas are recommended, several times a day with plenty of water. Avoid sweets, sugars, poor-quality fats, and excess rich carbohydrates. *Caution.* Any pain, restriction of, or bleeding from urine require prompt medical attention.

URTICARIA. See *Skin rash.*

VAGINAL DISCHARGES. Yeast infection with itching, offensive odor, mild inflammation, and white to yellow discharge. Herbal medicines: pau d'arco, goldenseal, pulsatilla (homeopathic), echinacea, garlic; also acidophilus. External: calendula or St. John's wort tincture or lotion; diluted tea tree oil, with caution on broken skin. Excess sugars, sweet drinks, dairy products, cold foods, fried foods, and junk food can make a person prone to discharges. Essential oils of chamomile, tea tree oil, or lavender, 8 drops, stirred into warm bathwater for a soothing, cleansing bath. Certain soaps, tampons, nylon underwear, tight polyester clothing, swimming pool water, scented toilet papers, and other articles may irritate the vaginal area. Prolonged use of antibiotics and other drugs can make a woman prone to vaginal infections. Herbs that are good for douches include pau d'arco, calendula, and goldenseal. *Caution.* Any unusual vaginal discharge needs a medical examination.

VEINS. Varicose veins is a condition that produces bulging, bluish veins. To improve circulation: increase exercise, lose weight if overweight, move your bowels regularly, and eat plenty of whole grains, fruits, and vegetables. Herbs include: gotu kola, ginseng, ginkgo, *horse chestnut*, and bilberry—recommended are the synergistic formulas. Topically: horse chestnut, witch hazel, or butcher's broom.

VIRUS INFECTIONS. Most viruses only become active when the system is out of balance, overstressed, and weak. If a viral infection is suspected, medical attention should be sought. Specific herbs: echinacea, goldenseal, St. John's wort flower top tea, olive leaf extract, red clover, schisandra, lemon balm, and osha. Herbal antiviral formulas can be purchased, as well as excellent immune-boosting combinations.

VISION. See *Eyes.*

WARTS. Garlic, bloodroot, or celandine juice; thuja ointment—all external use. *Caution.* With any color changes, bleeding, or sudden growth of warts—see a physician.

WORMS. Herbal remedies for pinworms or other worms should be administered by a professional, but three safe remedies that can work quite well are *garlic, black walnut*, and *pumpkin seed.*

SUGGESTED REMEDIES TO ADD
TO A FIRST-AID KIT

Arnica: ointment and homeopathic tablets (30x), calendula ointment, and St. John's wort tincture. Rescue Remedy (liquid dilution): flower remedy for emergencies to calm the nerves; echinacea extract. Tea tree oil. Ginger extract: for motion sickness, colds, and upset stomach.

TEN IMPORTANT
SYNERGISTIC FORMULAS

(1) Blood and lymph cleansing. (2) Energy boost. (3) Stress relief. (4) Anti-inflammatory (for the joints). (5) Digestive tonic. (6) Intestinal. (7) Colds and flu. (8) Allergy relief. (9) Immune tonic. (10) Women's or men's formula.

HERBAL

RESOURCES

American Botanical Council
PO Box 144345
Austin, TX 78714-4345
Tel: 512/926-4900
Fax: 512/926-2345
e-mail abc@herbalgram.org
www.herbalgram.org

American Association of Naturopathic Physicians
601 Valley Street, Suite 105
Seattle, WA 98109
Tel:206/298-0126
Fax: 206/298-0129
www.naturopathic.org

American Association of Oriental Medicine
433 Front Street
Catasauqua, PA 18032
Tel: 610/266-1433
888/500-7999
Fax: 610/264-2768
e-mail aaoml@aol.com
www.aaom.org

Herb Research Foundation
1007 Pearl Street, Suite 200
Boulder, CO 80302
Tel: 303/449-2265
800/307-6267 (to order only)
Fax: 303/449-7849
e-mail info@herbs.org
www.herbs.org

HERB SUPPLIERS

Blessed Herbs
109 Barre Plains Road
Oakham, MA 01068
Tel: 508/882-3839
800/489-4372
Fax: 508/882-3755

Eclectic Institute
14385 SE Lusted Road
Sandy, OR 97055-9549
Tel: 800/332-4372
Fax: 503/668-3227

Frontier Herbs
Box 299
Norway, IA 52318
Tel: 800/669-3275
Fax: 319/227-7966

Pacific Botanicals
4350 Fish Hatchery Road
Grants Pass, OR 97527
Tel: 541/479-7777
Fax: 541-479-5271

Gaia Herbs
108 Island Ford Road
Brevard, NC 28712
Tel: 800/831-7780
Fax: 800/717-1722

Herb Pharm
20260 Williams Highway
Williams, OR 97544
Tel: 800/348-4372
Fax: 800/545-7392
800/545-7392

Nature's Plus
548 Broadhollow Road
Melville, NY 11747
Tel: 800/645-9500
Fax: 888/665-0628

Rainbow Light Nutritional Systems
P.O. Box 600
Santa Cruz, CA 95061
Tel: 800/635-1233

BIBLIOGRAPHY

Hundreds of articles, magazines, journals, and books were consulted during the years of work on this book. The most important sources are listed here.

Beling, Stephanie. *Powerfoods: Good Food, Good Health with Phytochemicals, Nature's Own Energy Boosters.* New York: HarperCollins, 1997.

Bensky, Dan, and Randall Barolet. *Chinese Herbal Medicine: Formulas and Strategies.* Seattle, WA: Eastland Press, 1990.

Bensky, Dan, Andrew Gamble, and Ted Kaptchuk. *Chinese Herbal Medicine: Materia Medica.* Seattle, WA: Eastland Press, 1986.

Blumenthal, M., ed. S. Klein, trans. *German Commission E Therapeutic Monographs on Medicinal Herbs for Human Use.* Austin, TX: American Botanical Council, 1996.

Boericke, William. *Pocket Manual of Homeopathic Materica Medica.* Philadelphia: Boericke and Runyon, 1927.

Carper, Jean. *The Food Pharmacy.* Toronto/New York: Bantam Books, 1989.

——— . *Miracle Cures.* New York: HarperCollins, 1997.

Culpeper, Nicholas. *Culpeper's Complete Herbal.* London: W. Foulsham, 1952.

Duke, James A. *The Green Pharmacy.* New York: St. Martin's, 1998.

Felter, Harvey Wickes. *The Eclectic Materia Medica, Pharmacology and Therapeutics.* Portland, OR: Eclectic Medical Publications, 1985.

Foster, Steven. *Herbs for Your Health.* Loveland, CO: Interweave Press, 1996.

Foster, Steven, and Yue Chongxi. *Herbal Emissaries.* Rochester, VT: Healing Arts Press, 1992.

Grieve, Maude. *A Modern Herbal.* 2 vols. New York: Dover, 1971.

Griggs, Barbara. *Green Pharmacy.* Rochester, VT: Healing Arts Press, 1991. An excellent overview of herbal medicine in the West.

HerbalGram. Austin, TX: American Botanical Council and the Herb Research Foundation. A superb magazine about medicinal herbs.

Herbs for Health. Golden, CO: Herb Companion Press. Informative and practical.

Hobbs, Christopher. *Medicinal Mushrooms.* Santa Cruz, CA: Botanica Press, 1995.

Hoffman, David. *The New Holistic Herbal.* Rockport, MA: Element, 1990.

Holmes, Peter. *The Energetics of Western Herbs: Integrating Western and Oriental Herbal Medicine Traditions.* Vol. 1. Boulder, CO: Artemis Press, 1989.

Kindscher, Kelly. *Medicinal Wild Plants of the Prairie.* Lawrence, KS: University Press of Kansas, 1992.

Lewin, Louis. *Phantastica: Narcotic and Stimulating Drugs, Their Use and Abuse.* London: Routledge and Kegan Paul, 1961.

Lininger, Skye, et al. *The Natural Pharmacy.* Rocklin, CA: Prima, 1998.

Mindell, Earl. *Earl Mindell's Herb Bible.* New York: Simon and Schuster, 1992.

Newall, Carol A., Linda A. Anderson, and J. David Phillipson. *Herbal Medicines.* London: Pharmaceutical Press, 1996.

Pederson, Mark. *Nutritional Herbology.* Warsaw, IN: Wendell W. Whitman, 1998.

Physicians' Desk Reference for Herbal Medicines. 1st ed. Montvale, NJ: Medical Economics, 1998.

Rosengarten, Frederic, Jr. *The Book of Spices.* Wynnewood, PA: Livingston, 1969.

Shepherd, Dorothy. *A Physician's Posy.* New Delhi: Jain Publishing, 1983.

Teeguarden, Ron. *Chinese Tonic Herbs.* Tokyo/New York: Japan Publications, 1984.

Vogel, Virgil J. *American Indian Medicine.* Norman: University of Oklahoma Press, 1970.

Weil, Andrew. *Natural Health, Natural Medicine.* Boston: Houghton Mifflin, 1990.

Weiss, Rudolf Fritz. *Herbal Medicine.* Translated by A. R. Meuss. Beaconsfield, England: Beaconsfield, 1991.

Yen, Kun-Ying. *The Illustrated Chinese Materia Medica.* Translated by Nigel Wiseman. Taiwan: SMC, 1992.

ABOUT THE AUTHOR

Louis J. Vanrenen, one of the few professionals in the country with training in Eastern and Western herbalism, directs American Acupuncture, a holistic clinic in Boston. Over the last twenty years he has devoted his time to studying, teaching, and lecturing across the country about the value of homeopathy, acupuncture, and herbs, and the origins of Western and Eastern holistic medicine.